LIFELINES

LIFELINES

*The Intimate Experience of a
Transplant Patient and His
Family*

Ronald P. Jensh, Ph.D.

CONTENTS

DEDICATION

To those who cared
and
those who need care

Lifelines
accepted by ABC News for placement in the
"*Good Morning, America* Time Capsule 2000";
buried in Times Square, NYC 12/99

"I couldn't put it down"
"reminds us all of what it means to care for . . . patients"
—cardiac rehabilitation nurse

"I can't begin to tell you how impressed I am with it . . . I was moved to tears a number of times . . . an almost unbelievable example of the triumph of the human spirit"
—spouse of a patient

"a truly rare and valuable record"
"medical students are being made more sensitive to the emotional and spiritual needs of their patients through your (book)"
—minister

"words of encouragement as I faced the unknown . . . (my wife) was comforted and reassured by your words"
—cardiac patient shortly after bypass surgery

"(the book) will join our shelves with delight—we have no such information available"
—internationally recognized physician and CEO of hospital

ACKNOWLEDGMENTS

I would like to express my heart-felt gratitude to those who supported me and my family and kept encouraging us to continue to write and share our experiences. I am so grateful to my loving wife, Ruth-Ellie, without whose courage, love, and steadfast support I would not be alive. Special thanks are due to her for the long period of time she spent typing and editing this book, and for putting into print portions of my diary I could not relive at the time. To my two dear daughters, who have done so much to help and make the world so bright for me, my love and thanks for being who you are. For caring friends and relatives who offered assistance and prayers, and for so many students, friends, and colleagues who helped create this book through their suggestions and thoughtful critiques, my love; I am here for you, also. A special thanks to the medical staffs at the hospitals in Philadelphia which took care of me, most especially the heart transplant team, for all you have done. To Doug and Bob and Marshall, my eternal thanks for the many years of support and encouragement. To John, Perry, and the staff at 59 East, our deep appreciation for your friendship, the booth, and the coffee. All of you have been and continue to be my support system—my lifelines. I am here because of you; so I, too, can continue to be a part of your lifelines. My family and I wish to express our deepest gratitude to the donor family for providing the gift of life. I will strive to be a faithful and worthy caretaker.

God bless you all.

PREFACE

For the benefit of anyone fearing the onset of a heart attack, living through the trauma of its effects, or being close to one who has, we hope this account of a man who, at a very young age, had multiple heart attacks, triple bypass surgery and, much later, a heart transplant will provide strength, courage, and insight.

Reassurance is important to those who may face a similar condition. Surgery, when indicated, has been developed to the point where the odds are heavily in favor of a successful recovery. Knowing someone has traveled this road before and has recovered to the point of leading a normal life will, hopefully, lessen natural and sometimes overwhelming anxieties.

My family and I have met with over 1000 medical students, as well as critical care nurses and nursing students, patients, and patient families. We also have been fortunate to receive valuable feedback from those who read the original manuscript of this book.

It has now been almost eight years since the transplant operation, and much has happened in those intervening years. Distance in time has given me even more perspective on life and our abilities and responsibilities during the brief time we are granted the gift of life.

CHAPTER 1.

LIFELINES

Lifelines are those connections we have with each other which keep us alive, healthy, and in touch with ourselves and our environment. They are emotional, physical, and spiritual, and surround and encompass each of us. We do not have a single lifeline, but many lines coming from many directions and dimensions. They form a web upon which we are supported. We need only feel them and accept them—the choice is ours.

The source of emotional lifelines may be from within ourselves or from others. The internal lifeline is that self-determination to live, to fight; the "will to survive". It is the energy we muster in a crisis; when we refuse to quit and say we will "leave heel marks" if we are dragged out of this life. Not that we are afraid of death or the hereafter, but, rather, we are not yet ready to go and will fight to stay here for now. External lifelines come from family, friends, caring professionals, and even, at times, strangers who have that special quality of empathy. Language, actions, empathy and sympathy—all are a part of the external energy, as are loving words, written and spoken—all are lifelines. I felt that energy as a tangible force flowing into me and giving me the boost I needed to live following bypass surgery. It is as real to me now, almost 30 years later, as it was at the time I experienced it.

Physical lifelines are also internal and external. Internal lifelines refer to doing things which maintain the physical self. I had to alter my attitudes about my relationship to my body and how I care for it. I take care of my body for I am the caretaker of my self. The external lifelines are the physical support provided by others. Most obvious, of course, is the technical support from medical professionals. They have an ethical and moral responsibility to provide a lifeline; it is at the very core of their occupation. Family can provide extremely strong lifelines. During my crises my wife extended lifelines through embraces, words of love and assurance, and gentle touches. The energy imparted by touch can be sensed and felt; it is a presence. Others in my family, as well as friends, also provided important lifelines through their actions and words.

Finally, there are spiritual lifelines. For the spiritual self, the caretaker of the body, to be effective it must be strong. That occurs not only through ones own inner strength, such as the power of positive thinking, but also through strength imparted by others, often referred to as the power of prayer.

CHAPTER 2.

THE GAME

We are dealt a hand at the beginning of life and must proceed to play that hand to the best of our ability throughout the time we are allotted. The "cards" are the predetermined factors with which our existence is preset; genetics and behavioral characteristics passed down through generations, and the environment into which we are born.

Because of the experiences I have gone through, I have come to realize that these factors predetermined, in many ways, the direction my life has taken and were set more than a hundred years before I was born. Due to tremendous advances in medical technology, I have been saved from death time and time again. This has given me the chance to share my thoughts and experiences and, perhaps in some way, positively affect the lives of those around me.

My maternal grandparents were Victorian people, steeped in a northern European, English-Scottish background; stoic, unemotional. They did not openly display emotion, rather, love was expressed by providing the best they could for their children. Children, of course, were to be seen . . . not heard.

My father immigrated to this country from Germany as a teenager. His mother had died when he was little, and his father traveled the world as an architect. Coming from a country torn apart by World War I and then by civil war, survival was of utmost importance. There was no time for expression of emotions or personal desires, nor was anyone interested.

My mother later shared with me that, as a baby in the crib at night, I was left alone, crying a great deal, because it was time to go to sleep. I would rhythmically rock back and forth in the crib, a typical behavior pattern of children who are not obtaining their emotional needs. This, in turn, disrupted my parent's sleep and, at times, my father would tie me down so I could not rock. They knew no other way to deal with the problem. Today, the effects of early childhood experiences on adult behavior are well known.

My mother's idea of "motherhood" was an intellectual one. She was a highly educated, intelligent woman with a degree in theology. She simply had not been raised, herself, with the tools to know how to provide much physical or emotional support. She expressed this limitation much later in life when we talked candidly about the possible causes of my early heart attacks. She was very open and very honest, stating that she felt she was a good teacher, but not a good mother. She could intellectualize easily, but she could not emotionalize. I wish I had known at the time that she never attended the football games in which I participated in high school . . . not to deny me her support and pride, but because she could not bear to see me hit or injured. She internalized her feelings too well. As a result, my childhood lacked the physical and emotional support of my parents. As I grew up, I knew I was an emotional person, but I did not have the necessary role models to know how to express myself.

My brother's relationship with my father was openly adversarial for years. They had many loud arguments during my preteen years, and, as a result, I chose to be passive and compromising. I did not want to challenge my father because every time I saw my brother and father fight, they went upstairs and only my father returned. I understood this to mean my father won every time. Therefore, I could not go against an authority figure because I would certainly.

I should do all requested of me, regardless of my feelings or the possible consequences. Ultimately, I learned at an early age to internalize my emotions.

I always tried hard to please my parents; the authority figures. Yet I felt any attempt I made, school, sports, music, etc., as a youngster, was not good enough. This was never stated, but I interpreted their lack of support as my own failure to achieve. Today this family environment would probably be termed "dysfunctional". However, my parents were only working with the cards they had been dealt, and I do not "blame" them at all.

I pushed very hard during my Master's degree years. I could not ask for financial support from my parents since my brother had squandered his, and my father would not take the chance again. So I washed animal cages and flowerpots into early morning hours to survive. Professors were very understanding and helpful. Since there were no graduate student grants available at that time, marking exam papers and proctoring exams brought in occasional cash as well. But there was constant stress; physical, emotional, mental. This led me on the road to eventual catastrophe.

Ruth-Ellie and I met at the end of my first year. She was finishing her junior undergraduate year as a music major. We felt an immediate attraction. It was apparent to me from our first meeting that this was a woman of exceptional quality, and I wanted to know her better. The dating experience was very difficult for me, however, as I did not know how to react appropriately, emotionally, to another person. I had no self-confidence in an emotional situation. It was also a very stressful time for me, trying to win over this lovely young woman with whom I felt an immediate and deep emotional connection.

The dating time was blessedly short since we realized our love within three or four months. After six months we were engaged, and we were married two months after graduation. She was typically young and naïve, but she flourished in the marriage situation. We did not realize at the time, of course, how much she would have to grow; suddenly and much too young. She became very strong and matured rapidly as she took on the challenges we soon faced with a ferocity I had never seen in her. She was and continues to be the stabilizing influence in my life and the one I always turn to, as she turns to me, for guidance and support.

The graduate years as a doctoral candidate were a continuation of the stress I had endured during my undergraduate years, compounded by over-weight, smoking, and an improper but cost-effective diet. Marrying Ruth-Ellie was the brightness in my life; when I became unstressed was my time spent with her. Our time together was the only light I had, and this alone probably delayed the devastating events which would alter our lives forever.

As a result of my early experiences, I had become an obsessive-compulsive individual. I was a workaholic and displayed a typical Type A personality; the always-shaking-foot when sitting, the short, clipped speech pattern, the highly structured life, and the inability to be flexible.

Following my first heart attack, I had a lot of time to review my lifestyle and the factors which could have contributed to such a traumatic ordeal. There was no evidence of genetic involvement, so I turned to behavioral characteristics. Particularly obvious was my determined inflexibility and compulsiveness. Once a task was taken on it was to be completed at all costs and with no excuses.

I realized I had always been extremely competitive when I was swimming, and this was an area I could work on now. While doing laps with people swimming in lanes next to me, I would try to reach the end of the pool first. It was a driving force within me, even though everyone was there for the purpose of exercise and/or relaxation. They were not racing with me, but I made it a race in my own mind. Therefore, I decided to use my compulsive behavior to make sure I did **not** win! By consciously slowing down for several weeks, I actually conquered that compulsion and have used the same technique successfully in other areas.

Touching people was always difficult for me. I even felt uncomfortable holding hands with Ruth-Ellie in public. I had not been exposed to very much physical contact during my early childhood, and the fear of rejection was extremely strong. Therefore, I was socially very withdrawn.

As part of the enlightenment process, I began to make a point of touching people, using my compulsive nature again in a positive manner. A simple hand on the shoulder during a conversation was very difficult for me to perform, but I accomplished the "task" with conscious awareness, and ultimately the behavior became very natural to me and well received by others. Of course, these subtle touches are common behavior to most people, I later found out. With successful behavior modification, there was no longer a conscious effort needed, rather, the new behaviors became a part of me.

Stress, itself, is not bad. In fact, a certain amount of stress is good. It is how we deal with stress that determines the outcome. I did not deal with it well. I stressed myself unnecessarily and inappropriately and allowed other people's needs to become my priorities. I am convinced that my inability to handle stress appropriately was the single most important factor resulting in my cardiovascular problems. Again, using my compulsiveness to consciously delay accepting or completing tasks until an appropriate level of prioritizing occurred, led to a realization that there **is** a tomorrow and things **will** get done. There is not always only one right way; there can be many ways to do something.

For us to use the hand that is dealt us in life to play the best game possible, we must not dwell on what the hand could or should have been. We must understand there are many different ways of playing the game. We have the tools within us, if we give ourselves the time and motivation, to turn personal negatives into triumphs.

Unlike a game of cards, however, the game of life continues with the original hand we were dealt. The game is relentless, but, through self-awareness, self-examination, and constant re-evaluation of your position and choices, you can alter the way you observe the power of the cards you hold. Each new experience, positive or negative, provides an opportunity to reshuffle your hand to optimize and finesse your plays. As life draws to a close and it is time to lay down the cards, you can be confident you have played your hand to the fullest. You have won your game of life.

CHAPTER 3.

THE SECRET

The secret to a successful life is to set goals to achieve and hurdles to overcome. These are dictated by the expectation of society regardless of the reality of attainment. Once set these goals are to be reached or, better yet, exceeded. To fail at **any** task is unacceptable and will result in total personal disaster. Self image is tied to others' value of self. Therefore, you must always put forth maximum effort and achieve at the highest standard. Priorities society sets are good, right, and true, and you must adhere to them if you are to succeed and be admired.

All of the above are **WRONG**. All of the above are what I was taught to live by. All of the above are responsible in great part for the physical traumas I will describe. Only after I faced death did I start on the road toward changing my approach to life; a process which has taken many years and will continue to be a conscious effort for the rest of my life. Through will power and determination, and with the enduring love and support of my wife, family, and friends, I continue to fight and win my battle for self esteem and confidence. Attainment of goals is not the core of rewards in life. Loving interrelationships with and caring for people shines through. Life is the journey taken rather than the destination.

The best doctors attending the patient and most helpful people close to the patient listen. Then they talk. They try to understand the deep emotional feelings and needs of the patient. I was not looking for a "soothing syrup"; only for the reassurance I needed to overcome the constant, nagging feeling I would never recover or resume a normal life.

To fellow patients, I want to reassure you that someone has traveled this road before. The scars from that travel will heal just as the scars on my body are healing. To caregivers, my wife and I offer understanding and insight for the important role you play and the support and care you need for yourselves. To physicians and hospital personnel, I hope you will better understand that technology without compassion is meaningless. Technology applied with compassion heals!

CHAPTER 4.

THE ONSET ·

My first heart attack occurred when I was 27 years old. Hospitalization at the time was quite different from today. There were no special care units for cardiac patients, and there was no special monitoring equipment available. You were treated like fragile glass: total bed rest for several weeks, then slow recovery for one month at home, then carefully controlled steps back to work over the next six months. Drug therapy consisted mainly of anticoagulants, and, if needed, antihypertensive drugs.

Being in a private, for profit, suburban hospital owned by several physicians, various cost-cutting procedures were in effect; not always within regulatory standards. One Registered Nurse (RN) was on duty at night and on weekends for the entire 60 bed hospital. All other staffing was Licensed Practical Nurses (LPNs), trained personnel, and volunteers. RNs served food, attended to the well-being of patients, and dispensed medications.

Due to the busy schedule, it is not surprising mistakes were often made. I had recently completed my course in pharmacology and was well aware of the drugs I was being given. On one occasion, when night time medications were brought in, I looked at the cup and realized the wrong drugs had been put in my container. What I had in my hand would have killed me. I called this to the nurse's attention; the correct drugs were substituted, but nothing further was said.

Smoking was allowed in hospitals! During the day following the heart attack, my physician came into my room, sat down on the bed, lit up a cigarette, and suggested I might consider cutting down my smoking a bit.

The second heart attack occurred one and a half years later and was psychologically devastating. After all, I had now changed my life. I had done all the right things. I quit smoking, lost weight, changed my nutritional habits, and altered my life style. I could not resolve why I had been "hit" again. It made no logical sense to me. Although I was a student in a graduate school at the nation's largest private medical college, I was so emotionally tied to the physician that we never even considered transferring my case. That was the type of psychological power by which some physicians controlled their patients. They created a dependency and insinuated that they were the patient's lifeline.

When our family moved to New Jersey, we changed physicians and transferred my case to the hospital where I was now a faculty member in the medical school. However, the deep psychological damage continued.

One of the standard ways to treat depression was through the use of drugs. Valium and other antidepressants were widely available. These were not guarded drugs and were freely prescribed for me. The physician recommended that whenever I felt "down" I should take a small dose of medication. As time passed, I began using the prescription whenever I felt the least bit "down". Then I started taking a second drug as well. By the end of the year I was literally a drug abuser. It was not uncommon for me to ingest three to six dosages of drugs per day to keep from feeling low.

One morning I woke up and, for reasons still unknown to me, realized my situation. I said to myself, "This is ridiculous! I must face the life I have and deal with it, or continue to use drugs and destroy myself". At that moment I decided to stop taking any antidepressant medications. Seventeen years later I found the bottles in the back of a drawer, about 200 tablets. I had forgotten them and how near I had come to self-destruction. I destroyed them with the emotions of a victor.

I constantly feared another heart attack. After all, I had done everything right before but that did not protect me. Why should I expect I would not have another one at any time? Any pain between my knees and my neck was suspect. Any discomfort in the chest area was a definite signal.

I developed a habit of rubbing the center of my chest with my fingers to check for pain. I accomplished two things by doing this: I created pain by constantly pressing on my sternum, and I created a dark stain on all my white shirts that no amount of detergent could remove. Sometimes I actually wore out the fabric. Ruth-Ellie, my wife, and I developed a euphemism for my behavior which we called being "body oriented". Over many months of constant use this phrase began to annoy her. It created continuous anxiety in her. I was unaware of this because of my fixation with my own situation. Finally, frustrated and angry, Ruth-Ellie burst out, "Don't tell me how you think you feel. If you are having a heart attack you will know it. Then tell me". I was stunned! I had to face my obsession. At that moment I realized how much I had compromised the quality of our lives. I never again referred to feeling "body oriented". I stopped the habit of feeling for pain. My stained shirts were tossed out.

It appeared I was progressing well. Only one person detected my inner turmoil. My mother said to me, "You look like there is a shade drawn across your eyes". Less than a year after my decision to face reality, the shade was gone.

Family life also changed. My wife had faced the real possibility of being a widow in her twenties. She now took charge of her life, for herself and her family. Even today, more than twenty years later, Ruth-Ellie can tell you where she saw the last blue and white "H" sign (hospital) on a highway. She still notes what channel the police are monitoring whenever we travel.

Five years later, I was rushed into the hospital with a third heart attack. By this time Intensive Care Units (ICUs) had been established. They hooked me up to a monitor, and I "coded" (my heart stopped).

Death is not always sudden. One often realizes they are dying in the moments before losing consciousness. When my heart stopped I was still awake. I could hear the cardiac monitor behind me as its beep suddenly became a single continuous tone. I knew in those several seconds I was going. I heard the "Code Blue" alert and held my wife's hand as a tunnel of blackness closed around me. I whispered the words, "I feel dizzy". I was revived quickly as an injection of lidocaine coursed through the newly implanted intravenous tube (IV).

Ruth-Ellie was brusquely told to leave the room. She was alone for a long period of time with no idea what was happening. Finally a physician rushed out of my room toward her and demanded, "What religion is your husband?". Ruth-Ellie told him, and he disappeared with no further comment. She was alone again. No one talked with her. No one reassured her. It is still a subject of much anger to both of us.

ICUs were a new concept. Staff did not know how to handle ICU patients. Mistakes were made. The ICU was a prison for me for about 10 days; a prison which unintentionally destroyed a patient psychologically. The rooms had no windows to the outside and no clocks. Lights were on constantly, dimmed somewhat only at night. Meals, primarily light broth, were brought three times a day. Radios, television, telephones, magazines, newspapers, mail, flowers, books—none were allowed in patient rooms. The rooms were designed with a windowed door and a large window facing the nurses' station, arranged in an arc so patients could not see each other but nurses could see in.

Of course, patients do die in ICUs, but there was no provision in the design of the unit for moving these individuals without passing the other rooms. Therefore, nurses came around and drew the shades on the door and window of each room. It did not take long for us to realize what was happening each time the shades were drawn. It would have been better just to wheel the bed out. Drawn shades accentuated death. How or why would remain a mystery to fuel the anxieties of those of us who were left.

Patients were allowed visitors, immediate family only, no more than two at a time, three times a day, for 15 minutes; a rule rigidly enforced. No other non-professionals were allowed in the ICU from the time you entered until you left. This certainly added stress to the family, as well, as many care-givers lived a distance away, and there were no facilities for their comfort if they had to stay between visits.

The unfortunate result of such a low stimulus environment was depression and, most important, time disorientation. The latter, especially, has been an effective technique used to psychologically break (brain-wash) prisoners. Patients needed a great deal of inner strength to overcome this atmosphere. It intensified the pressures of trying to cope with a critical physical problem.

Monitors were located on a rack over the patient's head. Usually the sound was left on, and, although patients could not readily see their screen, they could hear the monitor. Even without the sound stimulus, patients often arched their back to see the monitor. Soon a peculiar transformation took place. The monitor no longer was a machine to record your condition, but a machine to keep you alive. As long as the monitor was normal, so were you. As long as it was moving, you were living. I did not want to leave the unit. I needed this monitor to keep me alive. A room without a monitor was terrifying. How would I know I was all right?

The establishment of Intermediate Coronary Care Units (ICCUs) has helped alleviate some of these anxieties. The best help possible, however, continues to be psychological reassurance from the staff. Unfortunately, most physicians are not trained to be sensitive to patients in this area. The primary responsibility falls on the nursing and volunteer staff.

My fourth heart attack occurred seven weeks after my release. I had been recuperating at home with no physical or mental stress.

Fifteen minutes previous I had taken a garbage can out to the curb (a man must feel useful to some extent!). A few minutes later I felt that familiar, constant, constrictive chest pain. It did not ease. It did not disappear. I knew what was happening. My wife called for an ambulance and got a neighbor to care for our little girl (Vicki).

My mind started racing. I remembered that during the third attack my heart had stopped for two minutes, and I doubted I would last this time. But it would be my good fortune to have one of the best thoracic surgeons in this country with a dedicated and able team at his side.

CHAPTER 5.

AN AFFAIR OF THE HEART

This story was written by Ruth-Eleanor several years after the first heart attack. Beyond relating a very unusual event, the story describes the feelings of a young wife who is suddenly faced with the real possibility of becoming a widow.

Spring has always been our favorite season. As it approaches, the new sights and scents vividly portray a feeling of birth, of life and vitality. This was our third spring as husband and wife, and Ron was working feverishly to complete his doctoral thesis. I found it difficult to be without his company while he studied, but I knew the end result was well worth our sacrifices.

Every morning Ron commuted by trolley and subway to Philadelphia. For a month or two he occasionally mentioned slight constrictive pains across his chest while walking the eight city blocks between the subway and the college. Once or twice he had to stop walking to catch his breath. He was helping colleagues move office furniture during lunch time and imagined the exertion was straining his muscles. There was little or no time as a student to do much about physical fitness.

The completion date for Ron's thesis had been moved back, so there were approximately six months of research to be accomplished in two months. It was humanly impossible to produce a worthwhile thesis in the time now allotted. Even so, Ron always rose to challenging situations. This was indeed the most challenging so far, and he would not admit defeat. Also, as a graduate student he was not in a position to tell his superiors what could or could not be done.

On a Saturday afternoon in April, Ron was feeling unusually tired. The pains in his chest had become almost unbearable, and it was impossible for him to concentrate. His arms, too, felt extremely weak. Work would have to wait. For the first time in his adult life he felt a nap would help. All seemed peaceful, and I woke him a couple of hours later. He had not rested well because of the pains which were now more severe than ever. He continued to relax in an easy chair in our living room while I laid on the sofa to keep him company for a while.

The next few minutes seemed like an eternity. My first awareness of Ron was the sound of unusually loud and heavy snoring. I got up and looked over at him. His eyes were rolling in his head, and his head was tossing wildly from side to side. I was terrified. I didn't know what was happening—whether he was dreaming or suffering some sort of trouble breathing. I yelled his name over and over but there was no response. This was no dream—I was certain. I ran to the telephone to contact our physician, and, as I dialed, everything became silent in the living room. I could see Ron's head was motionless against the back of the chair. His arms and legs hung limp. I wanted to run to him as a burning fear of what I might find welled up in me, but reaching the doctor was crucial.

Neither of us ever had much contact with hospitals. We felt we were very fortunate. I was instructed to drive Ron to the hospital where the doctor was affiliated. An electro-cardiogram was ordered, and within a short time the test results revealed I had witnessed a heart attack. Ron was wheeled away from me. It was to be the longest four weeks of our lives. I never realized how much I loved Ron and needed his presence, or how much I relied on him until I was suddenly without him. We were both frightened. I saw Ron cry for the first time and suddenly felt closer to him than ever before. I knew the coming month would be a difficult test of my mental and physical strength. I felt so empty, so alone, and questioned how capable I would be to carry on. But seeing Ron's desperation and fear was the necessary incentive to keep my spirits up while I was with him and to keep me going while we were apart. Our unspoken fear was that Ron would not recover. I couldn't consciously face the prospect, yet it was a definite possibility we both realized within us.

Because Ron was alive when we reached the hospital, his chances for survival were great. Each subsequent day improved these chances, yet it was difficult to take solace in statistics.

It is hard to express the volume of thoughts which passed through my mind during that lonely month. I was suddenly faced with the reality of death as a part of life. I realized how tenuous life truly is and how often we take our lives for granted. We had been living **for** the future, not **in** the present. There were so many things we had looked forward to sharing once Ron's studies were finished. We were just reaching the point in our lives when we could begin to enjoy ourselves and feel we were contributing members of society. How fruitless our struggles would seem if it were to be all over now. I am not a very religious person, but I prayed with all my heart for Ron's recovery.

As Ron's strength did return and his condition improved, it was important for us to consider the possible causes of his attack. He was young, 27, an unlikely candidate for a heart attack. Many of the contributing factors were environmental. He was a heavy smoker, 40 pounds overweight, and had been abusing his body by sudden acute physical stresses. No known hereditary factor was present. I have come to believe that a great percentage of the problem was due to emotional factors. Ron is an extremely intense and strongly competitive person, yet outwardly adverse to situations involving emotional display or conflict. As a result he had allowed outside forces to set his goals and pace, but the challenge thus created was impossible to turn down. Our own modern world is causing us to move at a terrific speed. It is highly challenging. We can meet the challenges and reach our own goals if we are willing and able to be sensible about our pace. No one else can determine what this should be. Others can only give us incentives to help determine goals which are meaningful to us. We fall hard if we allow outside forces to push us beyond our capacity. The challenge then becomes that of confrontation with these outside forces rather than the healthy struggle to attain our own goals. Ron was pushing his mind and body beyond their capabilities to meet an impossible deadline of someone else's choosing. As a result the completion of his work was delayed a full year and nothing academically was gained by the struggle.

It was a revelation to each of us that we could feel so completely a part of each other—so interdependent. I anxiously looked forward to visiting hours each day, but it was impossible to know ahead of time what Ron's frame of mind would be. The new environment and regimentation of his life brought on a deep feeling of insecurity with its consequent psychological manifestations. His moods rose and fell drastically from one day to the next depending, it seemed, upon the doctor's visit, tests being taken, the weather outside, and the path his thoughts had followed that day. But my visits seemed to be a bright spot in Ron's life. We felt closer to each other than ever before, and now believe the whole experience created a bond between us which is greater than most couples feel in a lifetime.

An interesting phenomenon occurred while Ron was in the hospital. While some may doubt its credibility, we were deeply affected by the experience. Ron had been having difficulty sleeping at night, and was given a strong barbiturate in addition to his regular tranquilizing drug one particular night. A couple of hours later he suddenly sat bolt-upright, trying desperately to throw off the effects of the drugs. He had a strong feeling I had come into the room to see him and was in the hall waiting for him to fully awaken. Eventually he fell back to sleep exhausted. At home, I had gone to bed close to 1:00 a.m. and had an inspiration to try something I recently heard about in the field of parapsychology; that is, the ability of some persons to travel "out-of-body"—to transport themselves through the power of their mind to another location. I totally relaxed my body and began thinking intensely of reaching the hospital, mentally picturing myself traveling from our apartment to Ron's room. I envisioned Ron lying asleep in his bed and felt myself calling him, passing through the room and into the hallway. Ron told his roommate the next morning of his experience and was puzzled he had been able to shake off the drugs to such an extent that he could sit up and be conscious of his surroundings. When I saw him that evening I talked about my experiment. We shall never know whether it was a coincidence of thoughts or an actual case of teleportation. What does matter is the **possibility** of the latter. We feel stronger and more positive in our attitude toward the future with the feeling that if Ron were ever to undergo such a trauma again but not survive, there is a chance our love might transcend the barriers of death.

As Ron's strength improved each day, so did our spirits. The day I drove him home was sunny and warm. I felt as though he was made of glass and felt each bump in the road was magnified. He walked slowly to the door. Every few steps up to the apartment he sat down and rested. What really mattered was that at last he was home. For another couple of weeks he rested and gradually returned to work at a relaxed pace.

To limit the environmental factors, as insurance for the future, he has successfully given up cigarettes, and is consciously maintaining appropriate weight. The doctor recommended a program of walking and bicycling which we both enjoy. The key to our physical exercise is maintaining constant, low-level, gradually increasing stress.

I feel as though we have begun a new life together. We are stronger as individuals and as partners from this experience. Ron is a new person in his outlook toward life, in general, and I respect and deeply love this new person. We draw strength from each other and feel so much a part of each other's life. It seems appropriate now that all of this should have taken place in the spring. It is truly a time of rebirth.

CHAPTER 6.

THE MIRACLE

A series of events occurred which one may attribute to luck, coincidence, God: I believe the latter.

At the time of my fourth heart attack, the hospital had recently opened a second catheterization (cath) laboratory. The chief of the ICU was scheduled to be away and was due to see me in a day or two. However, he had finished his obligations sooner than expected and decided to check in where I was rather than going home. Since the older cath lab was not being used for a few hours, he decided to do the procedure on me right away. Late that afternoon I was taken in and watched the fascinating process on monitors which the physician had positioned for my convenience and interest.

Several hours passed while my wife and I waited for the results. Eventually it became evident I was in worse condition than they had anticipated. One artery was 100 percent blocked, and two others were greater than 50 percent. I had a choice. I could be operated on tonight (triple bypass) or, most likely, I would be dead by morning. Although this surgery was still considered somewhat experimental, we had to proceed.

The surgical staff had already finished for the day and gone home. Somehow each staff member was contacted and returned for my emergency surgery by 9 p.m.. The operating room (OR) was quickly prepared, and Ruth-Ellie and I were told the facts, the probable outcome, the anticipated future, and the possible complications and risks. I was sedated before surgery, but it was the most terrifying time I had ever experienced.

Immediately after an operation, one usually remembers only flashes of moments. However, I remember vividly, even now, the sight of my wife walking into the recovery room (like a series of snapshots) and can still describe my surroundings in great detail. But there is one moment, in particular, I will never forget. Late at night, I woke up in some discomfort between medications. The nurse who was caring for me wiped my forehead and held my hand. I know with absolute certainty today, as I did then, that I lived because of her. I hung on to her petite hand with all my strength, knowing absolutely that if I let go I would die; if I held on I would live. It was as simple as that. I held on to this lifeline and I lived. Human contact is life saving.

During this time I also felt power, personal strength flowing into me. I was receiving energy from outside—a force I knew I did not have myself. It was a spiritual presence from the thoughts and prayers of others. That presence kept me alive, sustained me, and gave me the strength to heal my body.

Two residents arrived several days later to remove the stainless steel stitches in my chest. These 20 or so wires were placed with their tips protruding about a half inch above the surface of my skin. As it turned out, both residents had been students of mine, so they decided to have a "race". One would start at the top, the other at the bottom of the string of stitches. The winner would be the one with the most stitches in his hand. I sat in a chair and braced myself. It felt like a torch was searing down my chest, and, within several seconds, every sweat gland in my body opened. They finished in less than two minutes, but I looked like I had just been hit with a fire hose. As the pain dissipated, we cheered the winner.

After moving to an un-monitored room, my lunch was brought

to me one day. I sat in a chair beside the bed and, as I looked at the food, I suddenly burst into hysterical, uninhibited sobbing. I had finally reached a point where I no longer had to maintain control of my emotions. Somehow I knew I could relax, and with that relaxation, and the strain of all I had quietly endured, the emotional dam burst and the flood waters cascaded. I cried for almost 25 minutes continuously, until there were no more tears. With that, a great weight was lifted and the real healing began. It was then I believed I would have a future.

CHAPTER 7.

DIARY ENTRIES (1972)

Although my diary has been kept for a number of years, following are excerpts from the actual passages I wrote during this particularly trying time, immediately preceding and following the bypass operation. They show the direction of my mind—my fears, my hopes, my new life as I saw it could be.

May 15: Suffered ischemia (lack of oxygen) on Saturday night and returned to CCU (coronary care unit). It has been seven weeks since the last attack (with resuscitation); four weeks at home. Initial shock was terrific. Physically I feel good, but psychologically it is a terrible blow. RE (Ruth-Ellie) is really doing a great job of holding me together. I don't know what I would do without her. Am greatly concerned about her and Vicki.

The cardiologist wanted to move me out of CCU today, but the Director said he wanted me here one more day. EKG showed no change, but we must wait for the enzyme studies to determine if there was tissue damage. My insecurities start coming back. We may have to miss the usual Cape Cod vacation this year. It's hard to cope with that as it has been my one hope. Maybe Indian summer vacation. I need to get away, once this is settled, of course.

6 p.m.: My dearest Vicki, You are now about two months short of your third birthday. I am writing this because I have a heart problem, and I want to say so many things to you now in case I cannot be with you in body (I'll always be there in spirit) as you grow older. I will need an operation and it might not work out. There are many things to say and somehow I can't say them all. To tell you how much I love you seems so inadequate. You have been the light of my life. I am so proud and happy to have a daughter like you. I have tried not to be a biased father, but you are the most positive child I have ever known. And you already know what to say to "turn on" daddy. I remember in the last month when, for no reason at all, you would crawl into my lap and "want song", which meant holding you like a baby in my arms and singing "Rock-a-Bye Baby". You know, the first time you did that I cried as I sang . . . and the next two times, too.

You see, this is the first time your daddy has had to face a life-and-death situation and he is very frightened. Your mother is just wonderful and I love both of you so much. I can't begin to tell you of all the great things we did together, but there are movies and slides which will help you . . . and mommy can explain to you.

I am crying as I write this, as I am truly frightened of the future at this point. I am saddest because I may not get the chance to see you grow up and be with you through all those important times in your life when we will need each other. But I promise you, if there is more to life than here and now, I will be with you. And mommy, who is as much a part of me as any part of my body, will be with you . . . her love and help and guidance can help you as much as it has me.

I envy your newness in life as compared to my possible near end. Use it; enjoy it. Never be put down if you believe you are right. Be strong and sure and confident. Respect your body . . . . treat it as your home, for you are tied to it. Love people and love life. Be curious and learn. Sometimes it is hard but you can do it. You are my hope and my future.

I hope you will have some memory of me for that is most important to me. Mommy will tell you of our good times . . . we had so many. I hope we can have more.

Your loving father (daddy), Ron

P.S. Nobody can say "Oh, Daddy!" like you can.

8:45 p.m.: RE just left. Boy does she give me a lift. Her positivism and strength help so much. In some ways I am so jealous of her health and freedom . . . but so thankful for it, as she is really stronger than I am, even before my "problem". Her whole life outlook is healthy. Her faith is incredible. That is what I need and she is giving it to me. With faith we may just make it through all this. I am still frightened and depressed, but her hope is a light to help me hang on.

All of a sudden I am forced to face a life and death situation and I don't know how to cope. I am being asked to handle something about which I know nothing—not in our family or in relatives. I find it hard to hold on. It is a critical test for me. I will need all the help I can get; from myself and others.

11 p.m.: Just got word. Will probably do cath on Wednesday. Open-heart surgery to follow immediately, if so indicated. Dr. S. was a student when I was. Answered all questions. Very low keyed— good for me. Operation sounds wild. Seldom re-operate. Has done over 400 (about 32 triple bypasses). Frightening, but better it should come fast, if it has to happen. I hope no one makes a mistake!! Dr. T., the surgeon, often puts in several bypasses for each block— even repairs ventricular aneurysms. It looks like my moment of truth is suddenly approaching.

May 16: (Last minute cath today instead!) Operation **TODAY**—schedule change. Cannot get to will, which is being drawn up by the lawyer. It is my wish that the will dictated to the lawyer be carried out as stated. (signed Ronald P. Jensh, May 16, 1972).

May 20, 10 a.m.: I made it through the operation!!! Surgery from 9:00 p.m. Tuesday to 3:00 a.m. Wednesday. This is the first time I could write. Many emotions to get down on paper . . . and thoughts. Must wait for now.

May 22, 10:40 a.m.: Strange as it seems, I find it more difficult to write and/or express my feelings now. I tend to break down at any emotional thoughts or expressions. It's like a great water tank ready to let go. I am upset (afraid, nervous) about the one thing that's keeping me from leaving CCU. My electrical system is still irregular with extra beats. The control over them has been variable. Everything else is so good, but without this system all is lost.

I have had everything, just everything, going for me, and now this setback. The normal CCU stay is three to five days post-op. This is five days for me and no sign of moving. Oh, I don't want to go until all is well. I want the irritable heart tissue to settle down to normalcy. This time around I am **not** fighting to get out or depressed because I can't. I am doubting again; beginning to, not loose hope, but not have the confidence I had in a new lease on life.

All this has to be said because this is the one thing paramount on my mind, but I must talk well to my parents. RE is the only one I can be really truthful with . . . even then sometimes my thoughts cannot be expressed. In addition, today dysrhythmias seem to be present, although beating has a good average; the timing between beats is now varying. This has also contributed to my negative feelings.

Frankly, they seem to have tried everything (reactions to various combinations of medications) and still no change . . . if anything, it is worse. I shall tell RE of my concerns, as I am again going to need her support. My God, what would become of me without RE? I don't worry about Vicki now . . . the home visit was what I needed. Right now it has to be RE and me (and sometimes me alone) facing these crisis questions. The operation has been so fantastic that to dash my hopes once again would be so costly. I would continue on but my faith in the future would be very limited, if any at all.

May 23, 11:15 a.m.: The erratic beats are still there, but they seem to be less so. Several other aches and pains, but I will have to learn to live with them. I believe they will be moving me to a general floor today. The irregularities will have to be dealt with in some other way. I am still feeling unsteady about myself and my capabilities—the fear of all that could happen, I guess. I want the faith so badly, but am afraid so much.

Generally, I feel very bright, though tired, as opposed to earlier this a.m. Related to being told I could move out when a place is found. These ups and downs of emotional levels are wearing. I wish doctors could be made more aware of the psychological as well as the physical needs of their patients. A problem that should be talked about more.

9:15 p.m.: Tonight I cried a thanks to God for my life. I need time to have faith in the future, but for now this is purely an emotional release. I hope I can live up to the reasons why I have been spared. I must work on what my life purpose must be.

10:30 p.m.: Music— "My Cup Runneth Over with Love"— expresses so much. I wish I had the words.

May 24, 11:15 a.m.: I feel really down today; almost fatal as if all this will end and I will die—as if there is no chance for me. I'm really scared. I guess it's because of coming down from the operation, of the stitch pain, of sitting and thinking, and of being so insecure of myself physically. Sometimes, like today, I don't think I am going to make it. Maybe also because I want to make it so badly, I am afraid to have faith; that, and two hospital stays in two months after five free years. I don't trust myself (body), or time, anymore. I just want to love and be loved . . . but I feel deep inside I have to do more since I have been given life. I need RE so much to help me believe in things and in my own future as a viable living "going-to-happen" thing.

May 26, 8:45 a.m.: Today not so good. Started last night with a bout of irregular heart beats after dinner. I still am in a slightly irregular beat state. This scares me so. But perhaps because of this; of being almost there, but still having one "small" (the doctors say) problem, that problem is accentuated all the more so. It is also an uncomfortable feeling, plain and simple. One that reminds me that things are off.

Without RE here to keep me thinking straight, I start a negative spiral. I am afraid to believe in the possibility that I am healed. Part of it knowing the surgery and how complicated it was. It is hard for me to believe all that was done to me—and that it was all done right.

Going home and then back to normal will be the most meaningful steps right now. I wish to God the rhythms would become regular. I know I am selfish and audacious to want it all. I should feel so fortunate to have survived at all—and in no way can I adequately express how thankful I am. I guess I really want to be able to predict the future 100 percent—that's me, after all—and turn my back forever on this heart thing.

The truth is, I can't handle it well at all, so I want to refuse to look at it. After all, that was my reaction to the chest pain—delay, avoid. Now I know I have the best chance ever, and I am afraid to believe. Life means so much to me now—the sensations of life—I am afraid to lose it. Yet I become so preoccupied with not wanting to lose it that it interferes with making the most of life.

May 30, 11:10 a.m.: This, if all goes well, will be my last full day here. Hopefully, 24 hours from now we will be on our way home. Much of the time around and immediately after the operation is getting progressively more hazy in my mind. Probably just as well, in case I need another operation. Now, all I want is for time to pass so I can go home.

CHAPTER 8.

THROUGH THE EYES OF A CHILD

This story, about a three year old's perceptions, was written 14 years later as part of a high school English class assignment. Almost a year after starting to assemble my diary notes, Victoria mentioned she had written this story two years earlier, when she was 17.

Although my father had three heart attacks previously, every time was different. They had occurred on August 28, 1965, March, 1967, and April, 1972. Suddenly, on May 13, 1972, when he was home recuperating, my dad felt the onset of another attack. My mom called the ambulance service. Knowing she needed someone to look after me, almost three years old at the time, my mom called to our next door neighbors. They were sitting on their back porch, and their little four-year-old covered his ears, innately knowing "Vicki's daddy" was going to the hospital again and might die. The Chief of Police arrived shortly before the ambulance and administered oxygen.

My father was admitted to the hospital. He was rushed into the emergency room and hooked up immediately to machines. He then went to the Intensive Care Unit (ICU) with my mom at his side, holding his hand. As they were talking, both heard the "regular beat" of the heart monitor become a continuous monotone hum, while my mom watched the straight line on the screen, knowing this meant my father's heart had stopped. My father had just told my mother he felt dizzy, then had passed out. Across the hall at the nurse's station, the cardiologist leaped over the nurse's desk, his feet were off the ground, and called a Code Blue. Code Blue signals a special medical team that someone's heart has stopped and to report immediately. At this point, my mother was asked to leave the room for what seemed to be an eternity. Luckily, my father already had an I.V. in his arm, so the life saving medication which would stimulate his heart into beating again could be administered immediately. Even so, he was technically dead for two minutes. As my mom stood outside of his room, the doctor asked what my father's religion was so he would know what minister to call. My mom was devastated.

On May 14th, I showed my first real emotions and understanding of the situation. I could not sleep. As I walked into my parent's bedroom, I saw our close family friend who was staying with us to help my mom in my dad's absence. She was in my father's bed. To me this meant my daddy was really gone forever. I crawled onto my mom's bed and sobbed my eyes out in her arms.

After these incidents, all within hours, my father rallied and was able to rest in the ICU with full intentions of going home soon. As the doctors monitored my father's recovery, they noticed his blood enzyme levels were rising, a dangerous sign. On May 16th, the head of the catheterization lab felt my father should be catheterized, and he could fit him in that afternoon. A cath involves putting a tube in a blood vessel to take blood samples. Then the doctor "squirts" dye into the vessel, through the tube, and into the heart. This process shows the condition of the coronary arteries, and how well the heart is pumping, on a television monitor. The doctor found one artery almost 100 percent closed with the other two more than 50 percent closed. It was determined my father would certainly die during the night if he did not have an operation.

The operation room team had already left for the night, but

they were called back from their homes for 9:00 p.m. surgery. Before the operation, my mother went to see my father, yet she could not tell him about the imminent operation for it could be a dangerous shock to his system. While the male nurses prepped my dad for triple bypass surgery, the operating team was getting ready to undertake a procedure which, at the time, was only ten years old and had been done only thirty-two times at the hospital. A leader in the field of thoracic surgery was available to perform the dangerous, tedious operation. As my dad was wheeled into the operating room, he and my mom held hands and parted with a gentle kiss.

At home, my mom, neighbors, a relative, our family friend, and I sat on our living room floor awaiting the phone call from the hospital saying my father was out of surgery. I was put to bed close to midnight, and at 2:30 a.m. the neighbors left. My mom gave up waiting and called the hospital at 3:15 a.m.. The nurse said my dad had just arrived in the recovery room, so the three weary and anxious but hopeful grown-ups rushed to the hospital. My mother even wore a lab coat to be able to get in right away.

My father's recovery was uneventful. Most of the pain of the surgery was taken care of by drugs. When the metal stitches were removed from his chest, my father felt intense pain. He described it as a hot, torch-like feeling. With my father fully awake, two of his ex-students removed the stitches, racing to see who could re-move them faster. The pain activated my father's sweat glands so, when the students were done, his chair and clothing were covered with perspiration. Because my father was and still is a faculty member at the medical center, I was specially allowed to visit him even though I was not yet three years old. He came home on May 31, 1972, only two weeks after surgery.

It was ironic that while my father was in the hospital he had listened to a local radio station. He loved the theme music, yet never knew the name of the piece. Once he returned home, he accidentally heard a vocal arrangement of the song which answered this perturbing question: "How Do You Mend a Broken Heart?".

The following extemporaneous comments were made by Vicki in response to questions from a class of freshman medical students about four years after my transplant. They have been transcribed here because they address issues which could be of interest to the reader.

Every time the phone rings my heart pounds. I realize now, deep down, I don't have to worry like I used to, but I still do. I do a lot of the cooking at home, and I am very conscious of what ingredients I use. Now, at 27, I am nervous for my own health so I am very careful. At night when I can't sleep and my heart starts to race and I have an anxiety attack, I wonder if he could hear me in the next room if I yelled. I don't know how realistic that is since I am very healthy, but so was he at my age. Now it starts to concern me for my own health; my own life.

I don't think I was the normal high schooler. I didn't sneak away behind my parent's back. I didn't go to wild parties. I was always scared he would have a heart attack while I was gone, and they would need to find me, and I would get caught.

I don't think I have really dealt with the transplant issue yet. Of course, I was older. I was returning home after a year out of college, and Libby was a senior in high school. I was the one trying to be an indirect caregiver to mom and Libby. Later, Libby was not home that much because she went to college that fall, so I took mom out to dinner a lot to make sure she was okay.

Now I don't laugh a lot; I don't cry a lot either. I don't cry about the real stuff. The first time I remember laughing out loud was three nights ago when Libby was home and she put on some big band music. We were dancing around and my dad was teaching us how to do the "Lindy", and that was the first time I laughed really hard in three years. I go out and have fun with my friends, but it is not the same kind of fun.

I was 23 years old, and I didn't know any of the terminology the doctors were using (this was pre-"ER"). They talked to dad as Dr. Jensh, and they talked to **us** as Dr. Jensh. They were saying "fibrillation" and "tachycardia", and I'm thinking, "What?". It was a panicking experience because they didn't talk so the entire family could understand. I think a lot of times physicians do that; they talk to the patient, if the patient is knowledgeable, and it doesn't matter who else is in the room. It's terrifying not to know what's happening.

We made a comment last night how lucky we are. We went out to dinner, and the four of us always like being together. I think a lot of it hinges on dad's health. We never want to be apart when something goes wrong; we have this close bond as a family. I think eventually we do need some family counseling, or something to work out some issues as a group and individually. But it is such a new thing, the tragedy of heart transplant patients, and it is something where there are not a lot of professionals out there who have met people with transplants or dealt with their families.

CHAPTER 9.

DIARY ENTRIES (1992-1993)

November, 1992: *Although things had been going well for almost 20 years, since the first of the year I had felt progressively less energetic. It was suggested I come into the hospital for an electrophysiologic study (EPS) to determine if the drugs I was taking were having negative side effects and if some of them were really necessary.*

This course of action seemed logical, so on Tuesday, July 7, 1992, I voluntarily entered the hospital for what was supposed to be a three day stay, two days to run preliminary tests and allow time for the requisite drug to be eliminated from my body, and the third day for the EPS, following which I would go home. No one told me what the EPS entailed. I thought it was non-invasive—was I ever wrong! Little did I know this was the start of an extended stay, including two major surgeries.

July 9: Well, it's been a long time since I wrote in this diary. But, here I am again in the hospital after a long time free of heart problems. For a number of months I have felt less energetic than I thought I should, so I told my cardiologist. He suggested it might be due to lowered cardiac output from the Norpace. To be conservative, he wanted an EPS done. I met with a specialist in this area last January. It meant coming into the hospital for about three days.

This morning they did the study. It was supposed to take two hours—it took five! During the study I had uncontrolled tach (tachycardia—an abnormal, extremely rapid heart rate) three times and had to be revived by electroshock. The results of the study are that I have a "sick heart" (yeh, surprise!!). They cannot induce tachs in normal hearts. Now I am on procainamide and must stay in an additional four days to be tested again. The idea is, hopefully, the medication will protect me. Oh, the test results put me in the "high risk" group—that's why the extra monitoring, study, and stay. If the drug doesn't protect (they feel it will slow any tachs), it may give me time to get to a hospital.

Perhaps I was unprotected all these years and was just lucky!— for 20 years? I know all this is for "worst case" protection, and I couldn't be in better hands. Still, that is the logical side. Emotionally, it is a downer to say the least. Now all the old thoughts come back. I guess even after 20 years those thoughts are still just below the surface.

Having died three times today, it reminds me how easily it can happen. And, because my life is so good—wife, family, work— I don't want it to end. I don't want to leave RE—we need each other—and Vicki and Libby. I love them so much.

I am disappointed, depressed, and concerned. But I must keep reminding myself this is the best place for me, and all of this is to provide the best medical protection possible for me. The depression is nowhere near that of 20 years ago, but it's bad enough. I certainly have more positive confidence, but I'll be glad when I am back home again—I said "when" not "if" this time—I suppose that's an important difference.

July 14, 10:50 a.m.: Had the second EPS yesterday. I tached out before they even started the stress part. Very depressing; lots of tears. One of the EPS people came in and explained the options:

1. Take a more powerful drug which has severe side effects over time. He felt if I was 90 years old it might be feasible, but I could have another 20-30 years left so the toxicity would mitigate against this choice; 2. Do nothing. Play the roulette game and go home and hope. A tach at home means death. Still, why go through all this and then do nothing. It is not logical; 3. Open-chest surgery (thoracotomy—and wrap the heart in an "electric blanket" with a defibrillator attached. That has risk factors, as do all operations of that type; 4. New (five years old) implantable AICD (automatic implantable cardioverter defibrillator) with a five-year battery in the abdominal wall and wires via the subclavian vein into the heart. Much less invasive. The problem is that it is a National Institutes of Health study at another hospital. The procedure is not released for general use yet. I would need to be transferred. Also, they would have to check on availability of a unit. Treating this way has a greater than 95 percent chance over two years; greater than 90 percent over five, the longest time of the study now.

So that's it! All the old emotions came back and things were bad for hours yesterday. I had to work all this out in my mind. We chose number four, obviously. Now I have to remain in the hospital until the operation—time frame unknown. I cannot go home as they want me monitored at all times. I will miss Vicki's birthday this Saturday—and vacation may have to be postponed—we'll see what happens.

I need to remember technology has advanced greatly since 1972 (no computers, no microchips, no technology). Also, this is elective—to buy insurance by using the latest technology available. Remembering everyone recommends this approach, and this could not have been done 10 years ago, helps. I now do feel very positive and only need to put up with being imprisoned here. My main negativity now concerns what I am putting my family through—still, the other side is that it does bring us closer together.

July 16: Wait and wait and wait. No word all day. Tonight a downer. Seems they are having difficulty finding an AICD. It may be some weeks yet. But they don't want to send me home.

They started me back on half dose Norpace. One possibility is to retest (EPS) to see if Norpace protects, although that is highly unlikely. That really sent me down; the concept of staying here, but more so having to go through another EPS, knowing I will face taching and need to be shocked back to life again.

I really fell apart with the news, but this is the hand I have been dealt in life and I must play it the best I can. Vacation canceled—there will be other times. A guest lectureship canceled in Philadelphia—rescheduled for November in the Poconos. So who knows. All could work out okay in the long run. I must be patient and positive—"This, too, shall pass".

Again, I feel the presence of so many supportive people going out of their way to help me through prayer, offers of family help, expressions of love—beautiful and overwhelming. I have tried to be patient, loving, caring and compassionate toward all I meet. I know the outpouring I am witnessing is genuine—there is nothing superficial or momentary. I am even more enriched and believe even more strongly that what I do and who I am does count. Honesty, caring, and allowing oneself to be vulnerable is the right way; notoriety and fame are like shooting stars, a bright moment leaving little behind and soon forgotten. No! Immortality lies in the minds of those who know and love you and continues as long as there is someone who remembers you.

July 23, 7 p.m.: This is it! and I am scared, frightened, and very upset. I was transferred here this afternoon and am now in ICCU. I said good-bye to RE a few minutes ago. She is such a support—yet these final hours 'til tomorrow I am by myself. I know it takes a toll on her and she will cry now—not with me. I know she wants to be a rock for me, but I can see in her eyes the same concerns and fears.

I go tomorrow for AICD surgery. I stand an 80 percent chance of it working. If not, then things get more complicated as they will have to do a thoracotomy—also a longer time in the hospital. Tomorrow and the next days will be difficult (if I survive), but the long term is what counts. I have episodes of crying; mostly when I think of my kids and RE.

8:30 p.m.: Had thorough history and physical. Beginning to settle—resigned to fate? Moments of panic and fear—tears, but trying to maintain control. People here are very supportive. Still, this you face yourself. How fragile life is! And what little consideration we give to that fact. How suddenly we can go from normal living to a fight for survival or worse—death! We don't think about these things—we don't relish life until it is too late for most of us. The suddenness with which all this happened is so stunning to the psyche. Emotions have to handle so much—so unanticipated. Well, tomorrow I become a "bionic man". But the power of prayer and positive thinking—all those people pulling for me, sending their energy my way, giving me power to survive and heal—I have faith that will help so much.

RE, Vicki, and Libby—my three stars in heaven—what can I say? Words seem so inadequate.

September 8: I am starting my sixth week at home now. The operation did not work out as hoped, so they decided to do a thoracotomy while I was on the table. The short operation became five and a half hours. I also arrested three times in recovery, but the AICD did its job. It is actually an improved model called a PCD (pacer, cardioverter, defibrillator), so it also controls for slow heart rate. I came home a week after the operation (7/31). Very happy to come home; very grateful I heal so well and so rapidly.

I have waited so long to write because my emotional response to the whole process was varied and confused. I didn't realize, even after 20 years, all the associated emotions were still so close to the surface. They rushed back rapidly the night before the operation and in the days that followed.

There is a positive feeling that I am so fortunate to have access to this technology, and I will continue to live. In living, I hope I will make the most if it—where it really counts—sharing myself with others. I will continue to tell my story to future physicians in hopes it will make them more compassionate doctors. I have suffered emotionally and physically, but in that "gift" of suffering I have grown to realize how much I value my life. I realize everyone values their own life as much. Therefore, I should value theirs as much as I do mine. With that realization comes an understanding that I should cause no unnecessary suffering to others. I must then put equal weight on sustaining and maintaining others as I do for myself. Along with this are all those people who made a difference through their actions and words of support—who expressed their love, care, and concern—all those who often did not know me personally but gave me healing strength. It is a very powerful thing if we are open to receiving this very important source of power and healing.

There are also strong feelings of "why me". Intellectually and objectively I know this is natural. We always look at those more fortunate than we (healthier, richer, smarter, more attractive, etc.); we seldom stop to realize how many look at us with those same feelings—often with a great deal of justification. Still, those feelings are there.

But for the first time there was something else—**RAGE, ANGER**. I have tried to understand where this came from. I think it is because I was given no say about what was to be done. During the bypass time I could say op or no op—not really, since the alternative was death. Psychologically, there seemed to be a choice. The closest feeling I can relate to is if this is what women feel about rape. Then I can, for the first time, deeply and personally understand. I had no choice, not even the pretense of a choice. The thoracotomy was decided and happened—and I was violated!

Others, in a sense, attacked and penetrated my body without my permission. Of course, I signed papers and gave legal permission. But so much was coming at me the night before the operation I had no chance to consider. I am talking about my reactions (emotional, gut, non-objective, illogical) to all that happened. The lack of awareness—the severity and invasiveness—all led to the rage. The lack of someone professional to talk to, except for the technical aspects of the operation, and, later, the healing process, may have led to this anger being unresolved. I needed someone who was involved in my case to sit down and ask, "How do you feel?", "Do you have concerns, feelings you would like to talk about?". All were helpful, professional, and informative—none provided time or opportunity for treating my mental self.

I lost the summer; lost Cape Cod for this year. My life will have just as much quality, but some changes will be made—to help **prolong** my life at full quality.

This "experience" also reminds me that as much as I enjoy work, I need to slow down a bit. Those around me have already warned me they will get on my case if I don't behave. So all in all, this is a positive step; a short time of pain for a long term gain. Is that faith? If it is, I choose to embrace it.

November 22: RE's birthday. Boy, did I give her a present!! Came in Thursday night. The PCD fired off on my walk; kept hitting me. Luckily I was close to home. EMT and ambulance arrived, and I took three more jolts on the way to the hospital (a total of 12 tonight). **DENIAL.** I had all the symptoms of congestive heart failure and ignored them all. I was so lucky—God must want me here. This could have happened during my two business trips this past week. I was suffering for at least two to three weeks with this. In CCU for two to three days and treated with lasix (pumped out four liters of fluid in eight hours). The most terrifying night of my life! Last night I was walking the halls, and the nurses chased after me as I was in tach. It lasted about three to four minutes. They recorded it, and I told them what was happening. Now on procainamide so premature ventricular beats (PVBs) are singles and doubles.

Put down yet again, at least psychologically. So now what? Another cath? Another bypass? I don't know, and it is not knowing that tears me apart. So many knockdowns—my self confidence is so low. Now we wait! I anticipate some complex days ahead. Holidays—don't count on them (that really hurts). I must concentrate on more good times to come later. I am keeping tight control on my emotions, although sometimes I loose it briefly. I **have** to keep that up. I will not give up—I have too much to live for! Nice happening—everyone came in to celebrate RE's birthday with me—wow, so meaningful!

November 24: Yesterday I had a "BRUCE" stress test with thallium analysis. Sunday night—much anxiety and afraid of taching during the stress test, plus what the result would show. RE so helpful with her thoughts and support. She suggested lots of ideas and positive concentration of body strength; mind and spiritual strength. I was happy with the test. All appears okay. No new damage. One more step to get dosage levels right to limit the PVBs. RE reminded me I am here for my own good and should stay here until I can go home with no concern. For me and the family, here is where I should be. I am resolved to go home when the time is right. A turkey (not me this time!) can be cooked whenever.

7:15 p.m.: EPS tomorrow morning. No time frame for leaving the hospital—all depends on results. Because of RE's rules for behaving myself, I feel much more at ease. I must take things as they come; maintain a positive attitude. We take the future as it is handed to us. Considering all the desperately ill patients I have seen here, I feel **very** fortunate.

NOTE: I left the hospital the night before Thanksgiving and was home through the holidays.

January 11, 10:30 a.m.: I started going in to work once or twice a week (sometimes coordinated with visits to the cardiologist). During one of the visits in late '92, the topic of my emotions came up. The cardiologist said I had a classic case of depression—inability to sleep, loss of appetite, loss of libido, highly emotional.

Last Tuesday morning I woke up feeling light-headed and un-comfortable. RE and I came in on the train to check with my cardiologist before going to work, got as far as the top of the first set of stairs at the station, and I knew (so did RE before me) some-thing was wrong. I sat down on the landing, RE called the Phila-delphia Fire Rescue Dept., and they took us to the emergency room. I had an atrial flutter/fibrillation. It took them a couple of hours to stabilize me, then to CCU. Wednesday they anesthetized me and cardioverted my heart to normal rhythm.

Dr. B. (psychiatrist) came to see me and recommended an antidepressant which I started. Saturday evening I was moved to ICCU (couldn't beforehand as the unit was full). I was due to go home Sunday since everything was normal. From Saturday evening through to now things fell apart with couplets of ectopic beats and a general instability. It may be the antidepressant has caused this, but we can only wait and see. I should say (and will) that even before going on the antidepressant, I have felt better recently than before July. People have remarked that I look really good, better than six months ago.

I miss and love my family and find it difficult at times to think about them without tears coming. I did think at one time that if I died it would make things easier on them. I mentioned this thought, and RE and Vicki came down hard on me. This is a selfish thought. Love and concern and all the history of us together means commitment to each other and any problem should be shared.

Besides, **I want to live**; those dark thoughts have no place in my mind—unacceptable.

Right now (11:35 AM) there are many ectopic beats, and I am most uncomfortable. I try to control my emotions so negative thoughts do not overwhelm me.

January 24: One week at home and now back in the hospital again. Just after midnight Friday I had a severe dizzy spell and the PCD fired. I had had several spells of light-headedness and five to ten minute tingling sensations from the waist down since 5:30 p.m.. But it was qualitatively different from being light-headed from walking or other activities. So EMT/ambulance came, and RE and I came back into the hospital. No further problems since then, but the question is where to go from here. Hopefully they will interrogate the PCD Monday and find out what happened. Then options will be discussed.

The firing of the PCD really brought in reality. Now I know it's for real. That's alot to deal with mentally. I will never know when or where it will fire again or how often. How badly does this compromise my life and those around me?

We all walk a fine line between life and death, but for most people that realization does not occur until something catastrophic happens to them or to a loved one. Perhaps it is normally part of the mid-life change. For me, I have had to confront this issue much before my time and have been forced to make many changes in my life.

Sometimes I wonder if there is a greater reason behind my continued survival (more than 25 years since the first heart attack). Is there a greater good? Is there still something I am here to complete—some task to perform—an example for others?

I now have a very peculiar attitude concerning the PCD; a love/hate, friend/enemy feeling. The love/friend part is because it has saved my life. The enemy/hate is because it is in me and could jolt me at any time. Actually, intellectually, I am glad to have it. My emotional self has these negative feelings.

And what about **QUALITY** of life? I have had to change life radically in recent months: dietary restrictions, no more alcohol, no driving (just after buying the kind of car I wanted—mid-life crisis and all), and loss of lectures and teaching (which gives so much meaning to my life).

I often talked in the past about quality vs quantity in life. Simply the latter is not good enough. Without quality, why bother? One is simply going through the motions of living, but to what really meaningful end. Now I realize that quality of life is not solely what you do for meaning and/or pleasure. Life, itself, has a level of quality. It is inherent in the very word, LIFE. So one does not start with zero quality. Rather, one comes to understand there is a "minimum score" already there when life begins. How you live your life, where you find meaning, how you determine what is pleasurable and rewarding—all are additional facets that increase the score. For some, the basic score that comes with life is insufficient. They choose to end their lives.

Where do we go from here? I can only wait and see what happens. But, with a family like mine for support, and a wife of unbelievable courage, I must believe that whatever turns in the road may lie ahead, all will work out for them and me.

January 25: Well, the results are in, and I am having a difficult time trying to understand how to take it. I did have tachycardia, and the unit did what it was supposed to. The electrophysiologist feels that to change medications at this time would change the entire picture and might actually put me at greater risk. So the thought is to send me home and see if/when the next one happens. If there are several months simple and uncomplicated, then okay. Otherwise, we must consider what options are left. My problem is, it appears I have run out of options.

January 27, 7:00 p.m.: Well, things have really screwed up. It looked promising for going home yesterday or today, but yesterday morning I had a dizzy spell. I lay down on the bed and a few minutes later I tached out. It happened so fast I was not aware of going out. I just woke up with an endotracheal tube down my throat, bright lights, and a half dozen people working on me. The unit did not fire at first because I kept going in and out of its threshold. Finally, while I was out, it went off.

Once I was reasonably stable I was shifted to Medical CCU, put on lidocaine and procainamide IV. Yesterday the PCD manufacturer's representative had come in, interrogated the PCD, adjusted the unit to pace at a lower rate, and lowered the threshold for tach. Now the doctors were conferring again, and, as RE and Vicki arrived in my room, they told us they were going to try the "big gun" drug (amiodarone). This drug is generally used with much older people since, at some dosage levels, it causes toxic side-effects, including fibrotic lesions of the brain and liver. They hope it will work on me to stabilize the arrhythmia's at a low dose. They are interested in a short term response. The drug has a long half life, so it will take a week to ten days to build up in my system.

I asked about a heart transplant. I know the odds are not particularly favorable, but I also know I am running out of options. Dr. B. said I am an excellent candidate. At least it would resolve the issue one way or another. I hope this new drug will work, but if I continue to have the PCD firing frequently, then quality of life will be so reduced that the transplant, even with all its problems and statistical probabilities of success, would be preferable. I am still doing well psychologically, which surprises me.

9:30 p.m.: Still in ICCU. I'm feeling a bit apprehensive. I had non-sustained tach which corrected. I didn't feel any problems but the monitor went off with a warning. It brought to mind the fact that since it takes amiodarone a number of days to build, I am essentially having the same drug "protection" as before.

So, I am not a happy camper right now. A loss of confidence. Until yesterday I was walking the halls at a good pace. Now I don't know if I should go back to Intermediate tomorrow—to start all over again.

I was very depressed and down between November and January. Why I should have changed in January to a positive "up" mood I don't understand—but I did and I still basically feel that way. It is the short spells of apprehension together with thinking of the future that can frighten me.

January 30, 10:30 p.m. I had an extensive talk with the intern about 15 minutes ago. She was very helpful describing what the PVBs and bigeminies are in relation to my particular problem. It was very reassuring.

I am still "up". I hope this medication will be the winning one. Only time will tell. So I will continue in the hospital for another week or so—whatever time is needed to resolve this situation. I love my three special girls!!!

January 31, 7:40 p.m.: Basically I am writing this to relieve anxiety. During my 7 p.m. walk, for the first time I felt unsure and light-headed. Not much, but it really scared me—enough to sit in a chair in the hall for a minute. I've never done that before. No alarms, and the monitor appeared okay, but with usual extra (paired) PVBs.

I still feel uneasy—probably anxiety. I don't know if I felt the momentary strange feeling and it was exacerbated by my fright (anxiousness). I am trying to bring myself back to normal thoughts. I need to gain some confidence.

It scares me to feel this way. I am trying hard to control my thoughts and mind. At times like these I wish RE was here to help me. She is **the one** who cares. I hope this feeling will end soon. I don't want to call home because RE has had enough: she doesn't need to have an additional concern.

Midnight: Talked for 45 minutes to RE—boy, do she and her voice lift my spirits. Will be calling her at 12:30 just to make certain she is able to start up the computer in the basement. I look forward so much to this extra call.

February 1, 7:10 p.m.: Various people came in today—all are so very supportive of me. My cardiologist sat here for a long time, enabling RE and me to ask many questions. He asked if anyone had talked to me about a transplant. We said it had been mentioned as "part of the equation", but nothing more. He felt the electrical problem has been a difficulty. Being on amiodarone long term would not be good because of the toxic effect. He said the five-year survival rate of transplant patients is better than 90 percent. The surgery is straight forward. Post-op rejection is the problem. Typically you are on cyclosporine for the rest of your life—but all the other cardiac drugs are no longer given. The major problem is finding a donor.

This puts a different picture in the problem. It is, in my mind, getting progressively more serious. It is finally hitting me just how tough a position I am in. I am so lucky to have RE and my daughters. They provide so much emotional support. I can really scare myself if I'm not careful. I don't want my life to end. Someone once said, the past has been lived so don't think about it; the future is unpredictable so don't think about it; today is what is happening so think about it today. I need to control my thoughts; otherwise, living in the "today" will be compromised and could become a living hell.

February 2, 10 p.m.: EPS tomorrow at noon. I'll be anesthetized, and they will use the PCD to test me. I do not feel anxious, except for the results to be good. Looks like a week or so in here if the EPS is okay. They want to wean me off labetolol. If that works **and** the EPS is okay with the amiodarone, then I may go home.

Spirits continue to be generally up. I am emotional and start crying if people ask me how RE is doing. She is my life, and right now her strength supports me. I know it is taking a toll on her, and I wish I could take away her pain, emotional and mental.

February 4, 1:35 p.m.: The test went well, I was told, and the electrophysiologist plans to remove himself from my care—a good sign. Dr. B. stopped by this morning. I may be going home today. He said there was no reason to stay in just to wean me off the labetolol. He and Dr. G. were to talk, and he would get back to me.

From what they said earlier, I expected to stay through the weekend. I am not certain whether I am ready to leave, even though I want to. I'd rather stay longer to be certain I have the best chance possible. RE also has concerns about me coming home. She has a number of questions she wants answered before I leave here. She has suffered a great deal and, I believe, has lost confidence in my health. She needs to be secure that everything possible has been done to insure my health. I certainly don't blame her—on the contrary, I also feel that way. The trauma we both feel from failure doesn't make it worthwhile to come home before it is time. I also have developed a sense of dependency being here. To go home, which emotionally I want terribly, is only okay if the medical picture is as good as possible.

Right now the most important thing is to be certain everyone feels as confident as possible in my ability to be independent before I am discharged. Until then I need to stay in the hospital, knowing that "This, too, shall pass".

9:15 p.m.: Feeling anxious. Some trigeminies according to the monitor—I'm not used to that. I don't feel PVBs or unusual beats, but I am feeling ill at ease. I think it is a matter of possibly going home tomorrow. Lack of self-confidence. I hope I am not too much of a burden on my family.

We all look for assurance that our life will continue to be good and rewarding and we will continue to experience things together. That doesn't happen, and it is only a question of when that change occurs. For many it is well into retirement years. At 54 years of age, I see people in their 70's who are doing well in their lifestyles. On the other hand, we don't look at those whose lives are compromised or even ended at a very young age.

So what does it all mean? It means unpredictable things will happen, and we will never know when or where. We must accept the unknown and not let it compromise our lives any more than necessary. RE and I will continue to face these negatives as part of our lives. But we will also look for and experience positive things as well. We can only do the latter if we are convinced we have done everything possible to take care of the heart problem. Then faith and confidence will come. It will take time. Love makes my life important to me, and I will continue to fight for life as long as possible. When my life becomes too compromised, and the lives of my family as well; only then would it be time to call it quits.

March 1, 3:20 p.m.: I have been home about three and a half weeks. No diary entries as the mood did not strike me.

A week ago we met with Dr. P., from the heart transplant team at a city hospital which specializes in this procedure. I will be going in for a three-day stay tomorrow to determine if I am a suitable candidate. Since all indications are that this is the only viable option, I sure want to pass the tests. If I am rejected, I feel they are saying "Just go home and die". There are so many people supporting me—I never knew I had so much love with me.

Libby got accepted to her first choice college. It takes the last of the major concerns off me. Now I know all will be all right should I not make it.

I will be "walking in the valley of the shadow of death" (Psalms) for a while, but I do it because I know there will be a better time to come. I have to live with that faith. The faith is sometimes questioned, but faith and hope are all we have. My life has been outstanding. I am not ready to give it up yet. People will see my heel marks if I do not survive because I **will** be fighting death all the way!

March 2, 8:50 p.m.: I am in the hospital. This afternoon (after long waiting) I had a right heart catheterization. RE kept me company. The procedure went well.

I am really beginning to feel as if this body is solely a place for me to live and be alive. It is, in a way, separate from me; from the spirit that is me. It's as if I dwell in this body, and for "me" to keep alive I should do all I can to keep my body alive and well. That's the best I can explain it.

March 3, 7:45 p.m.: A busy day! Morning—echocardiogram and planagram (for teeth). In the afternoon, psychologist, a 567 question psychological test, sociologist, transplant head of nurses, dietitian.

RE couldn't contact me to find out when to come in. The phone bell in my room was shut off! Finally she called Patient Information, and they contacted a nurse who came in and found the problem. By that time it was too late for RE to drive in conveniently, so it will only be the phone call tonight.

Much has come at me today. Mortality rates, operation procedures, diet, etc.. The book *Information for Transplant Patients* was given to me. I read it. It fueled the fire of anxiety. It became **real** today! It will have to happen or I will most likely die within a year or two. Transplant is the only viable route, even with all the possible difficulties associated with it. I am truly "walking in the valley of the shadow of death". It is real. I may die waiting for a transplant (60 percent of patients do). On the other hand, transplant means a major change in lifestyle and many possible complications which could lead to death. Still, if I want to live, transplant is my only choice.

I have cried—broken down—a number of times, especially when I think or talk of family (now I am doing it again). I value my family and my life with RE so much that I lose it when I think of it all possibly drawing to a close. I broke down with the sociologist when I had to talk to her about RE, Vicki, and Libby. I want more time with RE and with my terrific daughters. Yet I feel time is running out for me. I doubt myself and my future.

I have prayed to God each night. It is for guidance, not for life. Life here or in the beyond of death is not a decision for me to make; nor is it something to ask for or bargain about. What will be done will be done. I can only ask for guidance for RE and me to make the appropriate judgments and decisions. With all the life-threatening situations of the past eight months, at any number of times I could have died, but I was in the right place at the right time. RE and I can't believe all this would happen to us only to have it end now. It just does not make sense. We wonder if this is happening because I still have work to do here on earth. I guess that is faith, but I don't dare believe or rely on that faith entirely. I am afraid to be that confident.

Now I can say with certainty I have tried to be a good role model—for RE, my children, friends, co-workers, and students. Most important is that we have provided a good, supportive, positive family environment. I have tried hard to be a good father to my girls and a faithful, loving spouse for RE. I guess the importance is in the trying, although there have been moments when I was not all I wanted or should have been. I have led a good, productive, rewarding life (much thanks to RE), and, when everything is added up, this is most important.

March 4, 11 a.m.: I stayed overnight for a VO$_2$ stress test. At 10 a.m. it was canceled! So now I have to come back as an out patient. I didn't have to stay overnight after all. Oh, well, nothing to do about it. Again, I am powerless.

March 12, 7:30 p.m.: Major storm, biggest in years, due to hit Philadelphia tomorrow! Things have changed radically since I last wrote. I went back to the hospital on Tuesday for the stress test and did very well. Not doing well would have put me on the transplant list. Doing well means it is likely I will continue to be managed medically until things get worse. So it was good-bad news. It seemed they did not feel the electrical problem was serious, with the PCD and medications.

I was home Wednesday and had what I considered one of the most normal, positive days in a long time. However, at 1:05 a.m. I had an attack of palpitations. It was a slow tach, but it did not stop. It was not rapid enough to set off the PCD, but would not revert to a normal sinus rhythm.

RE called the cardiologist, and, after much discussion, it was decided RE should drive me to the hospital. No need for an ambulance. We arrived at the Emergency Room (ER) about 1:30 a.m.. They tried to revert the tach, but no good. Finally, after about one and a half hours it reverted by itself.

Soooo, I got to my room at 5 a.m.. Poor RE finally left about 5:30 to get sleep and leave a note for the girls. The head of the EPS came in to tell me they would test for tach this morning.

They came in with the result about 6 p.m.. Thank goodness RE was here. The news was not good. The test showed I was much more at risk than they thought, and they cannot protect at low tach. They talked with the transplant team.

I will need the transplant and will have to stay in the hospital until a heart is found. The EPS doctor felt it would be too risky to go home at this point. In a way it is good news since it will deal in one way or another with my problem—hopefully successful (RE would smack me for that negative attitude). Now it is a question of my heart behaving until such time as they find a donor.

The depressing part is the waiting! It could be quite a while. I am at the top of the second priority list (Status II). Therefore, if they find the right heart but there is someone it matches on Status I (someone in greater jeopardy), they get it. If not, they go to Status II, and I get it. Although I am frightened about my PCD going off, I have to remember it is there to save my life, and I am in the hospital for maximum protection.

I feel very confident this is the way to go, and once we pass through "the valley" our lives will be so much better. If something should happen to me, I know my family will be all right. It was meant to be.

Of course, from my side, I want to continue to exist. I can do so much to help others, especially future physicians (my students). But there are many ways I can serve whether I live or die. I can only put my faith in God; however it turns out it will be for the ultimate good. I leave myself in the hands of God. I have faith in an ultimate force and being that governs our lives.

RE and I look at this transplant as a very positive answer to many problems, especially our lives these last eight months. Resolution will occur shortly, and, I fully believe, for the best. I am concerned about lasting long enough to be able to have the transplant. But aside from that anxiety, I feel strangely up and anxious to have it done. This is going to be good and positive for me, RE, and the girls.

8:30 p.m.: Thoughts—sudden. Is this really me? Is this really happening? I feel disassociated from what's going on; this is me, but I am separate from it all. What I have gone through and all I have to go through seems unreal.

There are so many people praying for me and wishing me well. That is so important. I believe so strongly in that power. Also, I feel confident my life has been worthwhile and I have made a difference in people's lives, having been here, because of that support. That is most important—the only thing that truly matters.

March 15, 6:45 p.m.: The "storm of the century" hit on the weekend. I am very glad I was already here. If this had happened on Saturday I would not have been able to get here. I try not to think about my present situation or the transplant too much. I can't do anything about the future so it is unnecessarily depressing to let my mind wander in that direction.

RE brought Libby in today. It was good to see her. I know she doesn't really like to come into hospitals, but she did it. She is becoming quite the mature young woman and has been doing much of the housework for RE.

The transplant nurse coordinator called me Saturday to tell me I am listed as Status II. She said I should call her when I get home. Apparently they did not get the message I am not going home! I hope they straighten this out today. I mentioned this to my doctors and have yet to find out if the situation has changed. Yet again, I feel helpless and powerless—and it angers me.

March 17: The last 24 hours have been something else. Last night a second-year student stopped by, and we spent most of the evening talking. We were standing in the hallway when the PCD fired. I was in tach about seven seconds. I did not feel any symptoms, it just went off. The nurses came running. I was put on a bed and taken back to my room. I felt okay but had an adrenalin rush (fright) that took 20 minutes to go away.

Today was okay, but about 9:30 p.m., while I was sitting on the window seat in my room, I suddenly felt that rush of possible tach again. I immediately lay down on the floor. My nurse checked the EKG strip. There was no evidence of tach, but I certainly experienced that feeling. A student nurse, who had atrial fibrillation which was corrected by ablation, said she used to get the same feelings. Perhaps it was a series of ectopic beats, but it resulted in an adrenalin rush again that took time to go away.

These things are what wear me out emotionally. Waiting is the most difficult part. Writing helps. I desperately want to make it through this dark valley and have that second chance at life. All I can do is keep myself alive as best as possible. And wait and wait and wait!

March 18, 1:30 p.m.: I am having real problems emotionally. My cardiologist came in shortly after noon. My best bet is to be transferred to the other hospital today or tomorrow. Practically I know this is best for me, but the emotional impact has been a lot more than I expected. I could still be there waiting for weeks or months. Another step in the dark valley. I will adjust—I must adjust and try hard to think positive thoughts. Attitude is all-important. I know once I am on the other side of the surgery, and in the weeks that follow, all will be well. It's just that I thought I would be waiting here with all the love and support of my friends. Now I will need even more courage to wait in a strange place among strangers. It will be more difficult for RE to drive an hour every day to see me. God, give her strength for the days and weeks to come. I feel so alone at times. Thank goodness for RE and family—they are my anchor, my foundation.

10:15 p.m.: I was transferred this afternoon. Many nice people here trying to make me comfortable. The transplant surgeon came in. I guess I was too positive. He stressed that this is a very difficult procedure, and I could die during the operation or even post-op. He emphasized the seriousness of my condition. But, if I don't gamble I can never win, and RE and I have very positive feelings. I want to live—I will be fighting for life as long as necessary.

March 19, 1 p.m.: This morning a number of doctors stopped in to check me. Medications are being adjusted. I find myself easily crying if I think about being here. I just want to be "normal" like last year. I am becoming insecure as to my fate. I try not to think of the future, but my confidence in a positive conclusion (transplant) is shaken.

Now that I am here where the transplant will happen, the reality cannot be avoided. I guess to some extent I avoided or at least intellectualized my state. Now I must deal directly with the reality of my mortality.

9:15 p.m.: I have to write. I had about three "episodes"; that shivery feeling as if in acute anxiety, similar to when I tached in January. I know they have done everything they can at this point, so I become even more concerned about staying alive until a donor is found. It is hard not to think such thoughts. I also feel jumpy. Unexpected noise startles me, and I have a lot of PVBs and bigeminies. I had that feeling after a lot of conversation, which has happened before. I wonder if over stimulation causes such reactions in me.

March 20: I try not to think about the future. But it is hard, being in the CCU environment. Oh, people are really nice and caring and the unit is state-of-the-art. It opened only two days before I was shipped here. It is just that I am hooked up to monitors and intravenous drips and back into the normal hospital routine. I know this is the best place possible for me, but that doesn't take care of the emotions. By-and-large I am dealing with it. I really have no choice.

When we are young we think we are immortal (that's why we bungee-jump, climb mountains, basically take risks). As we grow older, with friends and family dying, we have to face death as an integral part of life. But even then we intellectualize the process. It is not until we face our own near death or serious health problem that we have to come to terms with death and all we believe it means.

Because I value my life, I don't want it to end. The more you value something the more you want to hang onto it. Right now I want to be able to hang on until a donor heart is found. It strikes me suddenly that the same is true for the donor. Someone who valued their own life has lost the battle. I can feel the hurt. I know the pain and suffering. It is then, at the worst possible time, the family must decide if their loved one will be a source of life for people like me. It takes so much courage. Yet that person, in a way, achieves a sense of extended life through the gift that saves others. My life may continue because of a donor's heart. I will have the chance to touch and affect other lives, and herein lies immortality—for me **and** my anonymous benefactor.

March 21: I am in an anxious mood. The fellow in the next room is going for his transplant. At 6 p.m., eating his dinner, suddenly it was time to go.

What got me nervous was talking to a recipient who is here for rejection, four and a half months since transplant. All the things he has to do. He had been in really bad trouble for five years and near death (cardiomyopathy, liver dysfunction, other problems). He ended up with a temporary heart-assist. Then, two days before the donor came in, he had a stroke. He remembers very little during the five-plus months in the hospital. Now has a six year old's heart. Except for rejection (his second) he feels great. He fought for life, and, at the "gates", he stopped and came back to life. Reassuring is the fact that, despite all the hell he went through, he still says with absolute conviction it was (and is) all worth it.

It does set up anxieties in me, mostly the realization there are so many people in worse shape than I am. I am going to have to wait in the hospital for a long, long time until my turn comes, but there is no other choice.

March 22, 7:30 p.m.: Fifteen minutes ago, as I was reading the paper and watching TV, one of the transplant coordinators came in and said, "We have a heart for you". Stunned, shocked, scared, crying—**THIS IS IT!**

I called RE and then talked to the girls to tell them I love them very much, and if things do not go well they will see the skid marks; I will fight like hell for life. A friend who received his heart three years ago happened to call to talk. I told him, and I heard his wife yell a cheer in the background.

RE will have some supper, make some phone calls, and then come back in. I probably will go around midnight. It is still unreal. I am trying to calm myself—watch TV, look at the newspaper, wait for RE. As I will say to her, and as I have written so often, I LOVE YOU, RE. I LOVE YOU VERY MUCH—as much as is humanly possible.

Vicki and Libby, I love you both and know you will be successful. I would not have asked for better daughters. MY ETERNAL LOVE TO YOU, MY DAUGHTERS.

MY LAST ENTRY AT THIS MOMENT—I LOVE YOU, MY LIFE, MY SOUL, MY RUTH-ELLIE!!!

March 26, 8 p.m.: WELL, here I am!!! This is the first time I felt like writing. The operation went very well, but I went back to the OR once more to stop a "bleeder". I didn't wake up until Wednesday at 6:45 a.m.. Had an excellent day. Little pain. Got moved to CCU Thursday, then up here to a regular floor the same day. Have a single room (naturally) and am full of chemicals. Slowly getting tubes taken out.

I hear my heart, especially when it is paced. I continue to look for PVBs, etc.. Just unsure of my heart. Hard to believe the PCD is out, and I have a normal 21 year-old male heart. Now I get nervous that it and I will not get along. Yet many have stopped in with reassurance. I will feel more confident with each succeeding day and increase in activity. People say my color is back, and my hands and feet are warm for the first time in a long time. I hope all continues to go as well.

March 27, 7 p.m.: It should be an "up" day. Most all tubes have been removed. I ate dinner in a chair while RE was here, but I have chronic back pain that will not quit. Also drugs may be causing some emotional reactions. I cried for the first time since the operation. I am just feeling down. The reality of all this is hitting home. It is hard to believe all is normal. I have alot of adjusting to do. Everyone says I am doing well. RE continues to be my anchor and support.

March 28, 7:30 p.m.: Today (and last night) has been tough. I just need to remind myself the back ache is temporary. The dosage of cyclosporine, immuran, and prednisone has been upped so some stomach upset adds to crummy thoughts. Also, emotions are at the surface.

Much to go, but I have to believe I have crossed over the major hurdle. Now is the adjustment to a new life style, with all the abilities and restrictions. Others do it—so can I.

Oh, I am transplant #330!!

April 16: I went home after 10 days. Something went terribly wrong during that time; severe weight loss, dehydration, electrolyte balance way off. So back to ICCU for about two days, then back up to a regular floor for the rest of the week.

In trying to correct things, they saw my blood glucose level was dangerously high (another worst case scenario?). So now I have to learn to be even more aware of my diet, to measure my blood glucose, and to inject insulin. For a moment I broke down and wanted to call it quits, but the alternative (death) is not a viable option.

So I carry on with hopes all will settle within the next four to six weeks. Everyone says that is the roughest period of time. I must keep the faith and know "this, too, shall pass". Life **will** be better.

During the ten days Ron was home, he could not maintain his weight. At a regularly scheduled appointment, after five days at home, attention was centered on post-op edema in his ankles. We were advised he should limit fluid intake and double his dosage of Lasix. By the ninth day, Ron was extremely weak, and his vision was becoming increasingly blurred. Vicki and I drove him to the hospital where we had to call for a wheel chair to get him to the doctor's office. An infusion of saline solution was administered, and we were told to take him home. By the following morning, Ron had lost a total of 60 pounds in the ten days since his release from the hospital. He was almost blind, his skin was like tissue paper covering his frail skeleton, and he was in a diabetic coma. I arranged for his admission at noon. His glucose level was 1081 (results of the office visit blood tests for this parameter could not be found), and he remained insulin-dependent for the next four months. We are still managing some residual electrolyte imbalance. Through all of this his "young" heart remained strong and steady, but the ordeal left a profound psychological impact on all of us! REJ

CHAPTER 10.

TO HEAVEN AND BACK

The following was written by Elizabeth, my younger daughter, as part of a high school English class writing assignment several months after the original EPS procedure. She did not tell me about this until I mentioned I had been putting the diary notes together as a book. The impact the event had on her was enormous—and I didn't know!

People never think it could happen to them, but they could be the next victim. People feel they can treat their bodies poorly, but in actuality, they won't get away with it.

Our family was always happy together—just the four of us was perfect. Nightmares had passed through our home twenty years ago when my father had his fourth heart attack and triple bypass surgery, and we always wanted to keep it in our past. Our luck ran out last summer, and our world seemed to crash down on us, parting us but also keeping us all together. Everything was coming at us at the same time.

Of course, I, being the youngest, had no idea what was happening. I don't think I wanted to know. All I knew was my father would soon go into the hospital and be tested for some reason. As I found out more, he had volunteered to be tested for some medication he had been taking which caused some problems. This would last only a couple of days. As the doctors stopped one medication and started a new one, they realized the problem was much more complicated. Testing the medicine was a horror for both my father and the doctors. He arrested three times, and by the third time he did not want to come back. He was in "la-la land", very much at peace and loved wherever he was.

My father would now not come home for several weeks as an operation was necessary for his survival. The doctor's plan was to place a defibrillator in his heart to shock his heart in case it raced too fast. It would also give him a brand new life.

Depression set in on my family and father. We wondered what would happen and if he would be too bored in the hospital. A machine for his heart was needed quickly from somewhere in the country because there were none in Philadelphia. As time dragged on the operation came closer.

Our entire family dreaded the day he underwent surgery, hoping and praying we would not lose the one person who is most important in our lives. Without him my mother didn't know where we might end up. The doctors placed the defibrillator on his heart, and as he was recovering he flat-lined again three times, but the defibrillator clicked in each time and saved his life.

My father was in the hospital for twenty-five days, and mentally, it was extremely difficult. All the bad thoughts had to be removed because he now was someone different. Love was sent from everywhere. The power of prayer and believing he was a strong man helped our family greatly.

Tears of pain were shed on my pillow every night before I went to bed. I felt helpless and wondered if I would ever see my father again. With my friends supporting me to be a strong fighter, I knew I would make it as my father did.

I now realize how lucky I am to still have my father around. He brings me much laughter, fun times, and loads of tears. This is what makes us strong. We have survived the best and the worst of times, yet I took his life for granted because I always believed he would be with me forever. Now that it was almost taken away, each day that goes by I am thankful to see his smiling face and big blue eyes looking at mine!

STAYING STRONG

This story was written by Elizabeth in 1995, three years after the event she describes, for a college English course. Once again, she did not tell me until she had completed her assignment. It exhibits yet another aspect of an adolescent's feelings through a family crisis.

The long, narrow hallway seemed even more extended than usual tonight. Dimly lit, only one light hung from the middle of the ceiling showing the way to the sixteen steps which led to the bedrooms of each family member. I walked up each of those stairs, thinking over what I needed to do to get ready for the following day of classes. Although I was only a junior in high school, I felt more stress than most eighteen year olds.

The moonlight shone through my windows, between the curtains that gave me privacy during the night. Moonbeams highlighted the furniture, placed carefully around my room, and quickly disappeared as I turned on the round light switch against the wall. Not knowing where to start, I looked around with a dumbfounded expression and then decided to clean up the track clothing lying on my brown rug from the day's meet. I was relieved to have finally had a rewarding day of running, but running well was the least of my worries. The crickets sang their harmonious songs along with the wind that blew through the trees, causing my curtains to blow open. Although it was a chilly November night, the breeze allowed me to snuggle under my blankets to stay warm when it was bedtime.

A piercing whistle suddenly echoed from the alley-way beneath my bedroom windows. My father was always one to whistle for my mother after his walk if he had found something interesting to show her. But somehow I knew this was not the reason tonight. I slowly walked down the stairs I had so recently climbed, anxiety coursing throughout my entire body. Holding onto the banister to support myself, my knees barely able to travel the short distance, I reached the dining room and turned right into the kitchen. The brown, wooden side door had been left slightly open this crisp November night, telling me I did not want to see what was on the other side. Making my way past the kitchen table, smelling the left-over aromas of dinner, macaroni and cheese casserole, I grabbed tightly onto the brass door handle. Opening it further seemed like a chore as it seemed to resist, protecting me from horror.

My mother's voice spoke softly to my father as I made my way past the screen door, shutting it quietly behind me so I would not startle them. I proceeded down the porch steps and next to my father who was lying on the ground. I realized right then my suspicions had been true. Now I must face what I had been hiding from for months. Although I felt helpless, my mother quickly ordered me to retrieve a blanket to keep my father warm. As I wrapped it around his frail, helpless body, my sister was instructed to call the paramedics. Our family had been aware of my father's worsening condition; the defibrillator on his heart was firing off, but now my worst nightmare was coming true. I watched it happen with my own big blue eyes; my father reacting like he had just been kicked by a horse in the chest, was doubled over in pain and conscious enough to feel every jolt. I jumped back in fear, startled at what was happening, and covered my eyes to protect myself.

I was quickly rushed into the house, turning my head back as tears flowed non-stop from my eyes, wetting the hair that had blown in my face from the wind. Looking at the helpless figure on the pavement, I wondered if this would be the last time I would see my father. I paced back and forth from one end of the long, brightly lit kitchen to the other, my eyes still curious to see what was happening. Occasionally I peeked through the slit in the door, but I only saw black silhouettes highlighted by moonbeams.

My sister joined me and walked me to the front of the house

where we went past the front door and onto the large screened-in porch. Red lights flashed with eerie rhythm against our house; my eyes stared intently at them, and my ears listened to the worried voices of the paramedics. The words were not clear, and I wondered why my father was not in the ambulance yet. Holding me up with both of her arms, my sister tried to answer my questions and calm me down.

I stood on that dark porch, feeling alone as I had never felt before, wondering how long it would take them, and thinking it was taking much longer than it should. Only about half an hour had passed when the street became quiet again. Red lights and sirens faded into the distance as the ambulance drove off with my mother and father inside. Lonely and scared, I laid in my bed, waiting for the phone call that would determine our future.

Not until months later did we finally realize what was needed . . . a transplant. Once more, scared, alone, and afraid to tell anyone, feeling as if the world was a black hole and I was lost inside, I found out the procedure had been a success. It was as if spring had started early, and the flowers had begun to blossom after a harsh winter. Yet, as each day passes, I learn how important it is to communicate and show my fears, aas well as not taking life for granted; as quickly as I came into the world, I can disappear from it.

The following extemporaneous comments were made by Libby in response to questions from a class of freshman medical students about four years after my transplant. They have been transcribed here because they address issues which could be of interest to the reader.

I always wait for a phone call. I am always after him to see that he eats correctly and doesn't drink alcohol. I watch him just as much as my mother and sister do because he is so close to us.

I wrote my story in college when he had his defibrillator, during the night of the 12 episodes. My way of handling it was avoidance. I didn't talk to anybody and I still don't talk to anybody. I write a lot about it. Nobody really understands what it is about, and that's very hard because I am not open to talking about my family in that respect. None of my friends have been through it, so they do not know where I am coming from. When I do talk about it, it is really hard. Like Vicki, I don't laugh that much either. I think that is basically because I just shut down.

I noticed many of my high school teachers treated me differently because they found out what was going on at home. I guess they thought my grades might drop. They looked at me differently and avoided the topic. They just had their eyes out for me.

You find out who your real friends are when you need to talk to somebody, even if they don't understand. But I don't think I will want to talk about it. At college, my way of dealing with it is to hang up pictures of my dad. Any pictures I have of him I just kind of stare at. People don't really understand, so they ask a lot of questions. I don't know if I really need to talk. I think it's therapy for me to just write and keep it to myself because, in my view, nobody really understands.

CHAPTER 11.

CAREGIVERS

Caregivers are often forgotten in the rush to aid the patient. Therefore, we felt it would be most appropriate for Ruth-Ellie to write this chapter herself, as she has been my caregiver throughout these medical crises for more than 30 years.

Caregivers have an entirely different set of psychological needs which must be recognized, including understanding and support of their extraordinary responsibility. They need to be kept informed, to be pro-active in asking questions and receiving answers, and to be an integral part of the decision-making process. The medical community has yet to fully address this area, although indications are that awareness is now present, and some progress is slowly being made.

Communication is the key. Do not keep what is happening to you a secret. Talk about your concerns and fears. Talk to relatives, friends, physicians, clergy—whoever makes you feel most comfortable; whoever provides understanding and compassion. Many times I found I was not alone in what I was going through. Others had been there before who could offer support and true empathy. It is always important to have your feelings validated, whatever they are. Confront the situation head-on and acknowledge the importance of your role. Only then can those who would become your support system, your own personal lifeline, be truly effective.

We desperately need support, in many different ways, and must let people know how important they are to us. Never be afraid to ask for help or to receive it.

It may become quite a revelation to discover who you can really count on; who your true friends are. For one reason or another, some people cannot seem to face tragedy, in their own lives or anyone else's. Even the closest of friends or relatives may distance themselves when you need them most. Let them go and be thankful you found out—time is too short to be wasted tending a garden which will never flourish. The seeds of beautiful new friendships will be nurtured, and tightening bonds may be cultivated with some who had not had an opportunity to become as close before. It makes most people feel good and useful when they are allowed to assist in making the bumpy road a little smoother for you. Embrace the outpouring of their love and concern, and let them support you.

Small acts of kindness can mean so much when there are not enough hours in the day, and no time at all to do anything for yourself, alone. A dear friend supplied me with train tickets, while another took our trash cans to the curb for collection, and still another brought a meal which could be enjoyed without preparation whenever the girls and I felt like eating. One friend left cups filled with wild flowers on our doorstep.

As I stood in front of our house early one evening, trying to sort out the information explosion of the day and combat the numbness which was overcoming me in the stillness of approaching night, a tall, slender figure came toward me. Without a second thought, his gentle voice said, "You look like you need a hug", and he wrapped his strong arms around me. For that moment in time I, for a change, was upheld and supported, both physically and mentally. This wonderful individual was not a close personal friend, but a caring neighbor who sensed a need even I had not realized and reacted with sensitivity and compassion. It was a small act of kindness, but one of unimagined importance to me.

Laughter is as important to your physical and mental health

as are tears. Finding humor in some of the day's events or remembering something that brings a smile (perhaps a hearty laugh) is not irreverent. In fact, laughter can promote the healing process for everyone—it is good medicine. The tears will come— sometimes for no apparent reason or because of something inconsequential at the time. They, too, are part of the healing process. Allow yourself to grieve, even if only for the situation in which you, yourself, have been placed. Take time to be a little selfish!

If you have others, such as children, who need your attention as well, the process can seem overwhelming. When Vicki was little, we were fortunate to have wonderful, trusted friends who offered to care for her while I was at the hospital. Thanks are not sufficient for these important acts of kindness. Vicki seemed too young to be able to comprehend the upheaval in our lives. I am sure she was deeply affected, emotionally, but I tried to keep our home atmosphere as stable as possible. Eventually, both girls grew up knowing about their dad's medical history, and, in 1992 they were old enough for us to be supportive of each other. Luckily I discovered that Libby, the more withdrawn of the two, had not let her teachers know the trauma which was occurring in her life. I spoke to her high school guidance counselor who notified the faculty immediately. Use the support network available through the school system at every level, if it is appropriate. The staff can be watchful and supportive of your child, and know how to foster a compassionate peer group.

Caregivers can find themselves on an emotional roller-coaster. Daily changes in the diagnosis, the prognosis, the psychological mood of your loved one, the treatment received from your support group or the professionals in charge, even the weather—the con- stantly shifting "highs" and "lows" can be more wearing than the physical tasks you are now being called upon to perform. At times I welcomed a phone call or two from genuinely concerned indi- viduals who wanted to keep in contact and offer support. But many times I was truly angry, feeling as though my privacy and what small amount of quiet time I had for myself was being constantly invaded. I was forced to repeat the day's happenings again and again and listen and respond pleasantly to well-intentioned advice. I almost felt challenged to keep the news coming; if I could not provide excitement they would lose interest.

I have experienced the gamut of emotions, from intense anger, through hurtfulness and aggravation, to utter numbness. These feelings are natural. Nothing you **feel** can be "wrong", and no one can tell you how you **should** feel. I used to rely on such outside assessment, but it can be devastating to mind and body. Come to terms with your own feelings and personal needs so you can more fully understand your actions and reactions; to people as well as situations.

At times I actually wished (not prayed!) it would all be over. But, until now, that was a thought known only to me and God. I felt that Ron, especially, and our little family, too, had been through enough. Perhaps it was time to stop fighting. It takes great energy and courage to continue a long battle, but the final decision usually is not ours to make. So we keep fighting because our love is strong and the survival instinct is powerful. I certainly hope, however, I would be strong enough to support and defend my loved one's decision, should the circumstances be different and the pain too great to continue.

As a caregiver, you require a lot of inner strength (physically and emotionally) to be strong and supportive for your loved one. They can be **very** demanding without meaning to. Not only is your visit probably the most important part of their day (there are a lot of lonely hours spent in those busy hospitals which allow one's inner thoughts to run wild), but the incarceration can leave them feeling dependent and very vulnerable. They must be able to assert themselves somehow (not with hospital personnel, of course), and you are the easiest and safest means available to them. In your role as their advocate, you need to be aware of their needs and desires and be sure these are known and met. Put their mind at ease, as much as is humanly possible, and act on their behalf.

Of great importance, if at all possible, is to be available when the doctors are scheduled to see the patient. Your loved one is at a high emotional level, and there is tremendous room for misinterpretation. Ron often heard what the physicians said as depressing news, but I could ask them questions objectively for further clarification at the time or explain to him later what they really meant when he expressed confusion. During one visit in particular, Ron had "heard" he was given a 20% chance of living. When he repeated this to me that evening, having allowed the information to weigh on him terribly, I was able to remind him I had been there, and they said a 20% chance of **mortality**. I often wished for a day I could spend at home, but, because Ron told me know how important my visit was to him, I only missed seeing him two days during the year and a half of hospitalizations beginning in 1992 (one due to the blizzard; the other when the bell on his phone was inadvertently turned off).

Ah, yes, the bell on his phone had been turned off for the previous patient and never checked again! Ron kept leaving messages telling me he was in his room, looking forward to my call and anxious to know when I would be coming in. But it was a day of testing procedures, so each time I called back and got no answer I believed they had surprised him with yet another test. Once I finally reached Patient Information, and someone was willing to contact his floor, the problem was discovered and corrected. But **never** an apology—to me or to Ron. There was no apology when the wrong drugs were brought to him in 1972; there was no apology for medical mismanagement more than twenty years later.

No one is expected to be infallible, but we found so many times that staff and physicians alike are reticent to admit a mistake or error has even occurred. They stand behind their clinical shield. Do not allow the medical establishment to intimidate you. They often feel threatened, themselves, by an intelligent caregiver. Be assertive; be pro-active; be certain all of your questions are asked and you understand the answers. When you have a gut feeling something is wrong or needs to be addressed, act on it. Otherwise it can tear you apart inside for a long time, and you are not, in effect, taking good care of yourself or your loved one. You are a guardian and a facilitator, and you can work miracles. Have faith in yourself; know your rights; trust your intuitions.

Many times the medical community in general, specifically physicians, seems to have "bought into" its own importance far too much. We have tremendous respect for their knowledge and technical abilities. In most cases, without their expertise we would not be here today. But too often they display a lack of compassion and a distinct inability to communicate, with their patient as well as their colleagues. For example, we received the devastating news from one team of doctors that it was too dangerous for Ron to leave the hospital until a donor heart was obtained (it is not unheard of to wait more than a year, **if** the patient can last!). Shortly thereafter we were off-handedly told by another team's member we would be contacted at home when the organ was available.

I will always wonder why we were not told about the invasive nature of the EPS procedure. We were informed only that it was a simple three-day stay in the hospital. It would not have taken long to describe the nature of the procedure so we could be fully informed and mentally prepared. We also would have been able to take important steps for the protection of our family finances. Years before, we both had wills drawn up. However, it was not until **after** Ron's resuscitation from the EPS procedure that important documents, thankfully not needed, could be prepared. A notary at the hospital eventually witnessed the signing of our Living Wills and Powers of Attorney (so very important in the cold light of day), and I asked Ron to sign a handful of blank major medical request forms.

There was a lot of paper-work and a myriad of information to absorb when Ron was transferred to have the PCD implanted. However, I will never forget one resident's comment as he sat and gently spoke to us the night before the operation, "So they left it for us to tell you what's going to happen? We're used to that."

Again, we had not been fully informed in advance. We had relied on professional opinion and left decision-making to the experts. We were very trusting.

We are still trusting, that is part of "the power of the white coat", and, of course, they are truly the experts in their fields, but we now know the importance of asking questions, getting answers, and letting it be known that we are actively involved and require inclusion and consultation in the decision-making process whenever possible. It is most important to be informed of any alternatives available in the medical management protocol. With today's technology, it is not uncommon to avoid invasive procedures and their associated risks.

I was recently asked by a freshman medical student if the worry is over now. For me, **never**! Ron's health problems have been a major part of my life for over 30 years. With the new heart functioning so well, I might now change the word from worry to watchful, but there are still so many reminders of our tenuous situation, and old habits do not disappear easily. Whenever we travel I still keep track of signs indicating hospital exits, as well as local cellular phone numbers for emergency aid. I used to know all the warning signs so I could act fast. But the new heart has no nervous system; there would be no chest pain, no constriction. Except for statistics and clinical test results from time to time, I have no warning signs to watch for…I must rely solely on our communication and my intuition.

We should always be aware of the wishes of our loved ones regarding their treatment during catastrophic illness or injury and their disposition at the time of death. Our family has had many such discussions in the past; we feel the earlier the better. It is sometimes an uncomfortable subject to address, but it certainly does not have to be depressing. In fact, everyone's mind may be put at ease. Although the prospect of death to many is distant and frightening, we are becoming more and more aware that cessation of life can bring great peace and relief. It may, as well, be a beginning—not an ending. But peace and relief are not necessarily felt, of course, by family and friends.

Recognition must be given to the most difficult decision a caregiver may ever have to make. Tragically, too often a young life ends prematurely and powerful decisions must be made with great haste. It must be a terribly difficult time for any caregiver to issue directives—to suddenly determine what should be done in the midst of shock and grief. But the gift of life was given by such a family to Ron, and perhaps a dozen other recipients, when the empty temple of their young son was donated selflessly and lovingly. We have tremendous respect for that family and are doing everything we can to show our appreciation of the importance of their gift; to touch as many lives as possible, to treat others with compassion, and to offer understanding and support wherever we go.

Caregivers are an important part of the team which upholds the patient. Our role is essential to the healing process. Yet, at the same time, our own health can be put in jeopardy by the very acts of love, dedication, and self-sacrifice we perform. Be sensitive to the signals your body sends you; whether you are in need of rest or nourishment or a change of scenery, take care of yourself. This includes mental health as well; do whatever best relieves stress for you and be receptive to what "sounds" good; make time for yourself and never allow guilt, self-imposed or otherwise, to undermine what you need.

Lifelines must intertwine among the professionals, the patient, and the caregivers, and part of the healing process **must** incorporate physical, emotional, and spiritual support for the caregivers. Our contributions need to be recognized and our remarkable healing powers acknowledged and respected. Our active and positive role helps to make the miracle happen.

CHAPTER 12.

THE ROLE OF THE PHYSICIAN

During the acute repair process, of necessity, the patient turns over decision-making and self-rule and learns helplessness. I was put in this dependency role many times as a temporary measure to accomplish the physical repair of my body. But patients must be weaned from such dependency and allowed to struggle back to self-determination and control of their lives; a second, and essential part of the healing process. If this does not happen, not only is the "contract" with the patient not fulfilled, but, in fact, this omission contributes directly to the patient's decline, regardless of the level of technical support provided. Releasing patients without allowing and encouraging them to become independent is morally and ethically irresponsible. I have seen physicians who actively encourage that dependency, presumably to inflate their own egos or because they want or need to maintain control, perhaps due to a sense of inadequacy. In these instances, maintaining patients in such a state is reprehensible. More commonly, doctors are just not sensitive to a patient's needs; an unfortunate situation, so easily remedied, which compromises the patient unnecessarily.

Dignity is easily stripped from the patient during prolonged hospitalization, and with that can come a profound loss of self-respect. If not recognized and addressed, it will eventually compromise the mental healing process which, in turn, will compromise physical healing.

As a professor teaching medical students, I especially stand in awe of the diagnostic and operative skills of physicians. But I have come to realize the great need for consideration of the patient's feelings. The mental condition of a patient, if not positive, can undermine recuperation from the most successful surgery. Surgeons apply themselves to their immediate task but often give little or no time to concern for the patient's mental status. But after surgery the patient needs the most help, mentally and physically. There are constant doubts and worries about the smallest feeling of something not being 100 percent normal; the nagging discomfort, the worries of things imagined or real as you lay alone in your bed. Our health care professionals must be trained to relate in an appropriate manner to their patients. Otherwise an adversarial relationship can develop—the antithesis of what should happen. They need to know that competence and compassion are both essential qualities in providing the best health care possible. These components are not mutually exclusive. It is also their obligation to assure not only that they, themselves, act accordingly, but that their colleagues do as well. I have had the privilege of teaching more than 5000 medical students since my bypass operation and have tried to be a positive role model for them in all areas.

I am absolutely convinced that touch is an essential part of the healing process. It is a form of non-verbal reassurance that has an enormous impact, more so than words. Making physical contact indicates to the patient that this is their time: I am here for you; how can I help you? The extra time spent by the physician is insignificant. I have come to feel, many times it is not that the physician heals patients, but rather the physician helps patients to heal themselves.

There was a period of time when physicians were trained to touch a patient only when they were performing a procedure or examination. Otherwise that was violating personal space. Toward the end of the 60's and early 70's, a change was initiated, not surprisingly, within the nursing profession. Nurses provide the majority of physical and emotional patient support. Medical students, by and large, are rarely trained in this area during their clinical years. Physicians need to look at the patient not simply as a machine. Too often they try to repair the "engine" without knowing on what "model" they are working. Physicians must look at the whole person in their treatment paradigm.

As I look back through all of my hospitalizations, I am struck by one major problem which stands out far above the others. Physicians are well trained to address the health problems of the patient regarding the identification and treatment of a disease state. However, they are usually poorly trained in dealing with the patient as a person or providing the kind of emotional support the patient often desperately needs. Training is similarly weak in understanding the fears and concerns of the family. I was fortunate to have experienced some very caring, supportive, and dedicated medical professionals. But in our fast-paced world, where patient contact time is minimized to maximize profit, skills which may have been learned often are not used. I would like to share two examples which demonstrate a profound lack of concern. The first is a general scenario I experienced, which occurs all too frequently; the second is a specific situation which happened to me.

Hospitalized patients are usually involved in a serious, very personal health problem. They are anxious and concerned about their condition and what will happen to them. They have about 18 waking hours to think of questions to ask and thoughts to express when their physician arrives. However, when the physician does come in, a quick physical examination is generally performed and several cursory questions are asked. The doctor is there a matter of minutes and quickly moves toward the door, displaying an anxiousness to leave. Seeing this, the patient often becomes too agitated to even remember the questions, conceivably elevating blood pressure levels as well. Thankfully, there are those physicians who ask a patient if they have questions, then wait, perhaps sitting or standing near the bedside, betraying no urgency to leave. A gentle hand on the arm or shoulder of the patient can work wonders, too. Time lost to the physician—at the most a few minutes. The gain—probably a faster and more complete recovery.

In the second case, I was in the intensive care unit when the director and his entourage of residents arrived at my door during rounds. Before entering, they stood in the hallway to discuss my case. I watched the entire animated discussion through the large window, although I could hear nothing since the door had been shut. As the group finally entered, they surrounded my bed with the director on my right. On my left was a particularly vocal resident. While they listened to my heart, the resident stated indications were I that was in an irreversible condition and would probably die, according to an article in a recent cardiology journal (they forgot I could understand their scientific jargon!). The director disagreed, stating that in this case it was probable there would be an uncomplicated recovery. They continued to argue over me for many minutes; death to my left, life to my right. I was watching a tennis match and was very anxious to see who would win! But they left and took the game with them—unresolved in my mind; unfinished; terrifying. These professionals had forgotten where they were, and egos took to battle. How uncaring; how cold; how unforgivable. Yet, technically and tragically, all was being done in a professional manner, and "education" was taking place!

The true "team" approach to health care may evolve into the kind of support system which is so desperately needed by the patient's family, and we have been fortunate to see it in action. A team of physicians generally refers to one or more "group practices" working in concert with each other. Perhaps this is necessary because doctors have become so specialized in recent years, or possibly the threat of malpractice looms too heavily over their heads. But the heart transplant "team" incorporates the fields of discipline we have long felt would be appropriate in many situations to best serve all of the needs of the patient and family alike. Nurse coordinators are available 24 hours a day to listen to concerns, answer questions, provide explanations, and act as liaison between you and the doctors, as necessary. They are knowledgeable in all aspects of the pre-and post-transplant process and serve as expeditors. A member of the psychiatry department is on hand for emotional needs of the patient and family members. A social worker offers additional support and counseling in many areas from the formation of support groups to understanding insurance coverage (or lack thereof!). In addition to cardiologists and the surgeon, a dietician and physical therapist complete the team.

Part of medical school education generally includes lectures concerning management of a physician's office. This is a necessary part of the students' preparation to enter the medical world. Recently, however, major blocks of time have been devoted to discussions of financial incentives, investment opportunities, and programs concerning maximizing profit through manipulation of funds, use of accountants and financial advisers, and partnerships and group practices; how they operate to assure the highest financial gains for the physician. Although these are discussions of the realities of today's world, the issues often are presented as major considerations which imply to the student that they are of primary importance, often seeming to take precedence over concern for the patient. First year medical students have asked repeatedly, "How can we treat our patients with care and concern when we are told we must maximize the number of patients we see each day so we will be considered successful by our hospital or group practice?". After only six months in medical school, students already get the signal from their role models that their primary goal is to make money.

Our medical schools, either by implication or by unintentionally misplaced emphasis in the curriculum, are sending a strong message to students—a message which would horrify those who truly understand and remember the pledge they made as they received their diploma and entered this profession; "You will exercise your art solely for the cure of your patients" (Hippocratic Oath). The desire to be financially successful is a reasonable goal, but is totally unacceptable if it becomes the primary goal for anyone in this profession.

In social settings among physicians, seldom, if ever, are the concerns of patients, the philosophical determinants of medicine, or the best way to be supportive of patient family needs, discussed. Typical conversations revolve around the perceived success of the group practice, defined by yearly earnings. How soon one will have accrued enough money to retire ("the earlier, the better") is a major topic. Other topics include: are the bank charges for managing my pension fund reasonable; Medicare is ruining our profit margin; insurance companies are bleeding us dry; a good accountant/financial advisor is the most important asset I have; I can't make a decent profit. The country club's annual fee and the cost of golfing and travel are a real concern. Certainly not all physicians have lost their sense of perspective; not all have forgotten the meaning of dedication to their profession. But many have and more join these ranks each year.

Our medical schools are faced with an information explosion. The temptation, too often realized, has been to emphasize technology rather than interpersonal skills. The lay public progressively sees doctors as highly competent professionals, providing excellent technical support, but with a coldness and lack of basic understanding or concern for their patient's emotional needs. Our medical schools must not train a physician to be just another technician, doing a task, collecting a salary, and going home.

The practice of medicine is an unusual mixture of demands for it is the art of a healing science lovingly administered with humanity—it is about people helping people! Anything less should be unacceptable. The exceptional physician achieves the complete balance while maintaining a healthy personal identity in the process.

CHAPTER 13.

STEWARDSHIP

There is a definite responsibility related to receiving a life-saving organ. As recipient of this precious jewel, one has agreed to take on a commitment; a guardian role. That role must be consciously fulfilled to the best of one's ability.

It is tempting but irresponsible to try to continue leading one's life as if nothing has happened; to go on without regard to the quality of life or the need to alter one's lifestyle to assure the body and transplanted organ receive the best care possible. One cannot continue to abuse their body, but must address the factors which could have caused the original problem and be determined to do everything possible to protect the new life they have been given.

With unpleasant memories, I enter the hospital on a regular basis for check-ups and biopsies. The smell of disinfectant, the sterile atmosphere, the reminder that I must always rely on medications and physicians in order to lead a "normal" life...I approach each visit with trepidation and anxiously await the test results. Knowing how well I feel in general, it would be so much nicer to put off these visits. But my responsibility is to my new heart, the donor, his family, my family, the physicians who performed the miracle, and the patient who might have received this organ had I not been fortunate enough to be selected.

We have seen some patients who have not attended to their stewardship role, and it is obvious they are maintaining the same lifestyle as before: some have not stopped smoking; some continue to drink alcohol irresponsibly. Perhaps most obvious is the lack of a significant behavioral change, demonstrated by their attitude, their demeanor, their approach to people around them. They demonstrate inflexibility, hyperactivity, and compulsive behavior. Many have retired, either from work or a productive life in general, and have withdrawn from society with a "sick heart" attitude. Their interests seem to revolve around comparing levels of medication and how much food "plants" (transplant patients!) need because of steroids.

A case in point was a patient hospitalized for rejection of his new heart. The rejection was caused, at least initiated, by a fight which this 40 year old man had while drinking in a bar and becoming irritated with another patron. In the course of the physical confrontation he was hit in the chest several times. It was obvious his lifestyle and behavior patterns had not changed. He was irresponsible, and he had ignored the responsibility he had to his donated organ.

Another part of the stewardship role relates to other people. With this new life comes an opportunity to change not only one's own lifestyle but the world as well. The additional time given should be used to do things of value to humanity: to give back; to make one's gift of life meaningful to others.

I won the lottery, but I cannot leave it at that; then the gift of life is empty and meaningless, and the giving of that gift is worthless. Each year I ask myself what I have done with the extra time granted me to improve myself, my relationship with family and friends, and the community. How have I changed, and what have I done in the time between when I died and now to affect people for the better? How many lives have I touched, and, as ripples in a pond when each pebble is cast, how many lives have they, in turn, touched because of me?

CHAPTER 14.

THE HEALING TIME

During the years following transplantation I have had the opportunity to spend brief times in solitude in two distinct areas of the country; the mountains of Colorado and the sand dunes of Cape Cod, Massachusetts. In these beautiful surroundings, I have meditated on how my experiences have changed my personal approach to life. These thoughts I gladly share with you in hopes that you may be enriched by the words.

In my youth, I exposed my body to many potentially de structive situations. I was young and immortal. But when you are young you do things like bungee jumping because accidents always happen to the other guy. At my age I say, "Hey that's a very exciting thing to do, but no way in hell am I am going to step into space like that."

I never had a "typical" near death experience, described by so many patients. With the PCD implant, I was simply not unconscious long enough, if at all. However, I recall quite vividly the time I experienced a very strong emotional reaction which many others have encountered. During EPS testing, when they had difficulty reviving me, my immediate and uncontrolled reaction to being brought back to life was rage and fury. I have never been as angry in my life as I was at that moment. They brought me back to this world, and I did not want to come back. I had been somewhere else, I know not where, but I was more peaceful and content; more relaxed; more warm and comfortable than ever before. I wanted to go back, and I was angry they had the effrontery to revive me without my permission. The passionate anger passed, but I will never forget that moment or that feeling.

For over six months following transplant surgery, and 30 pounds lighter, I put off buying any clothes to fit me. The expenditure represented an investment and a level of confidence in my new life I simply could not allow myself to make. I was afraid that buying new clothing would actually set me up for another disappointment, like a jinx; an illogical, totally emotional reaction.

It took over a year and a half to begin to have confidence in myself; in the "new" heart. For so many months I lived with all the phantom pains of my sick heart, firings of the PCD, old thoughts and anxieties about a heart that struggled daily, fears that any moment my new heart would malfunction catastrophically. But each year has been better, and the last two years have been the most enjoyable of my life.

Sometimes it takes a life-threatening event, hopefully just the natural aging process, to understand the body is a machine; like any other machine, but based on organic material. We live inside this machine, and the only way we can stay here is to make sure the machine is well maintained. Of course, this includes good nutrition, physical fitness, and a good mental attitude; whatever it takes to keep the machine in good working order.

Rather than fear, respect and sensibility are key factors in determining what we should or should not do with our lives. Skydiving is fine, but is it right for me? Should I take the chance? As one gets older one usually decides they do not particularly want to live on the edge. I have lived on the edge, the "cutting edge" of cardiology, long enough. I do not want to be first in line anymore; I have been first in line for intensive care units, for bypass surgery, and pretty close for heart transplants. Now I just want to be part of the crowd.

We all deal with two sides of our being; the intellectual side and the emotional side. Once a patient has been through a life-threatening situation, every little "abnormality" can cause a panic reaction. They want to run off and share with somebody close to them and be told everything is okay. It does not matter that I am trained in the field of medical education: I still do it. It is similar to well known instances of cardiologists who suffer heart attacks, go through denial, and end up hospitalized or dead despite years of clinical experience.

Traumatic, life-threatening situations are particularly difficult for men. In our culture, men are not trained to network; to develop a group of supportive people to whom they can talk freely, in a very intimate way. Women do this more readily and effectively, as they are generally more interactive on the verbal level. Therefore, men are, perhaps, more at risk.

For me the psychological damage has been almost unbearable at times, but I keep remembering how good the good times have been and that they will happen again. Each passing day heals and lifts me that much further from the nightmares of those dark and terrifying days. We must come to terms with what has happened and learn to live a fuller, more meaningful and vibrant life as a result. My family and I will be repairing our psychological lives for years, perhaps the rest of our lives, and we will never be the same. I am very fortunate to have three strong people who support and love me. It really allows me to carry on. Now is the true healing time.

I do not have to restrict my lifestyle unduly. Of course, I do not go cross-country skiing in sub-zero weather, but I never did that before, anyway. The key is to be aware of fatigue and regulate my activity accordingly. There are on-going tests, but I take fewer medications than I did during the two decades following the by-pass surgery. We continue to watch the statistics of transplant patients as each year passes. There is nothing I cannot do as long as I remain sensitive to the signals my body sends me. Regular moderate exercise and a healthy diet allow occasional excesses which provide added quality to my life.

That is not to say everything has continually gone well. I contracted hepatitis-C due to blood transfusions in 1972, and I became infected with CMV virus from the donor heart. This was quickly attended to, but later resulted in a detached retina and cataract. Eventually a lens replacement operation was successfully completed. Cyclosporine, the anti-rejection miracle drug, also creates its own specific side-effects with which we must deal on a regular basis.

Medical checkups four times a year, a biopsy every six months, and a right and left heart catheterization every year, in concert with other pertinent measurements, are constant reminders of my unique situation. I feel the Sword of Damocles always hanging over my head. But I am learning to believe again; to go from a weak-heart to a strong-heart mentality.

A new way of perceiving myself and the world has resulted from my experiences. I had always been taught, both in academic courses and through my religious upbringing, there is a duality to each of us. We are spiritual beings who dwell in a body; a machine or temple in which our spirit or soul resides. Body and soul must be inter-connected, of necessity, to "live" in this world, but the two are not immutably intertwined. The soul may leave the body, yet the "shell" as a functioning biological unit can be kept alive, as has been shown by our abilities to sustain a body although the person is "brain dead" (perhaps a euphemism for the fact that the soul has left the temple).

Following transplantation, I became truly aware of the difference between the temple in which I dwell and the self which I am. This leads to an understanding that dying is a process by which the machine ceases to function, but has little to do with cessation of the spirit. I finally understand the implications of this relationship. There is now a remarkable separation. I am fully and continually aware of my "self" as distinct from my body. I truly understand the difference. At times I actually **feel** this "duality". On numerous occasions, when talking with others, I find myself mentally "standing to one side", feeling the sensations of the moment and observing and evaluating my conversation simultaneously. It is as if I were watching the behavior of another person for that moment.

I am convinced by my own near death experiences, and those of others, that life is more than what our five senses provide. Physical senses help us to survive, grow, and thrive in the physical world. We are well aware there is much more to the physical world than we sense, as shown by studies with different animal models. They see, hear, taste, touch, and smell a world often entirely different from that which we sense. All are simply ways of sensing our physical surroundings. Senses are used to keep the body alive so the spirit (soul) can remain in this time and space.

At night, before drifting off to sleep, I pray. It is a kind of review of the day; what was successful, what could have been done better and how. Also in my prayers are thoughts of love and protection for all of my family and for friends in need. I think again of the preciousness of life. It is a jewel that is handed to us at no cost. We accept it very much for granted, and yet it is so fragile. We never really understand how wonderful life is, especially when there are bad times. It is a unique experience for all of us and it will not come this way again.

I thank God for allowing me the extra time to improve on my life and for giving me the tools to be sensitive to the needs of others and, hopefully, to be a better role model for others around me. This is not a time to make deals with God. It is not a time to wish for things. It is not a time to be superficial. It is a time to reflect and a time to try to remind myself how fortunate I am. It is a time to talk to God and to ask for the strength to be better tomorrow than I was today. I also add my thanks for the days to come, however many or few they may be.

There is a lot to be said for the old Golden Rule many of us were taught as children. However, perhaps it should say: "Do better unto others than you would have them do unto you." Try to be a better person: a more considerate person; a more sensitive person.

If everybody tried, this world certainly would be a much better place.

The spiritual world is a totally different dimension which we also inhabit. Advances in technology, which now allow us glimpses of that world, reinforce my conviction that this aspect of life does, indeed, exist. We have had faith through millennia that that aspect of ourselves exists as separate and distinct from our body. Many religions have spoken of the intertwining yet separate natures of body and spirit. We are just beginning to have the opportunity to "see" that immortal part of ourselves.

I have experienced a profound change in attitude and priorities, a personal and professional growth which has led to an entirely different way of teaching, of relating to people, friends and family, and of interacting with colleagues. I have come to understand it is the relationship among people that is important, not the attainment of goals. Too often we seem to be so busy we lose our sense of caring and compassion. We do not take a few moments to offer a kind word, or to support, or to listen. In our rush to accomplish a task we forget to be gentle; to be compassionate to one another; to be courteous. I still strive to attain realistic goals, but I have found it takes very little effort and less time along the way to show care and concern, and the results are so rewarding.

Hopefully, sharing our experiences with others may ease some of their pain, fears, and anxieties which are normal and faced by all who encounter life-threatening situations. I hope family members will better understand their loved ones and young men and women entering the medical profession will understand the necessity of ministering to all the needs of their patients.

All of my experiences, all I understand of life, now leads me to one inescapable conclusion; I do not live alone. I am supported by lifelines from many sources which uphold, nourish, and guide me through this life. The wondrous part is that as I am nestled·in my own lifeline web, I, too, provide a portion of the web for each person I touch. With these inter-connecting lifelines we sustain each other and raise ourselves to new heights of understanding and compassion for all mankind.

The healing continues . . .